It's *Good* to be *Here:*

Stories We Tell About Cancer

David Giuliano

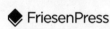 FriesenPress

Suite 300 - 990 Fort St
Victoria, BC, V8V 3K2
Canada

www.friesenpress.com

ISBN
978-1-5255-2712-8 (Hardcover)
978-1-5255-2713-5 (Paperback)
978-1-5255-2714-2 (eBook)

1. BIOGRAPHY & AUTOBIOGRAPHY, PERSONAL MEMOIRS

Distributed to the trade by The Ingram Book Company

Dedicated to those who are weary of the battle.

"We are each one of us parables."
–William Stringfellow, 1982

Table of Contents

Preface

Stories: That's All We Are

"It's good to be here." Whenever I'm asked to speak publically, that's how I like to start. I wish I could remember it at the beginning of each and every day. I've been treated for cancer on and off for more than twenty years. To paraphrase Keith Richards, the hard-living co-founder of The Rolling Stones, it's really good to be *anywhere*.

And it is good to share some stories. I share them to remind myself of the small miracles—the precious slant of afternoon light, the sound of a prayer, the attentiveness to beauty—that illness awakened in me. I share these stories hoping there will be redemption in the telling, for me and maybe for you.

In each of his 2003 Massey Lectures for the Canadian Broadcasting Corporation, Indigenous writer and broadcaster Thomas King began by saying, "There is a story I know." Then he would tell the ancient story about the creation of the earth on the back of a turtle. He concluded each telling of creation with: "The truth about stories is, that's all we are."

The stories we tell and are told create us—our identity, our culture, values, and worldview. They are how we make meaning of our lives and bring depth to our humanity. Stories can expand us or shrink us and the world we inhabit. If we are told as children that the world is a safe and beautiful place, it will powerfully impact how we engage it. The same is true if we grow up hearing that strangers are dangerous and not to be trusted. If we are told that we are good and kind creatures, there is a very good chance we will turn out that way. But the stories we're told can also bring us shame and destroy our souls.

In illness, the stories we tell and are told can bring comfort and insight. They can shape treatment and amplify healing. Over the past twenty years, and through multiple recurrences of cancer, I have heard and told many stories about illness. Some of those stories have been healing, others have not.

My medical condition is a two-word short story entitled: "Dermatofibrosarcoma Protuberans"—"DFSP" for short, because Dermatofibrosarcoma Protuberans is a long, boring, and for all but the clinically inclined, incomprehensible story. It is recorded in digital databases and on clipboards. Its plot is a marathon of surgeries, radiation treatments, climbing blood pressure, strokes, and medication. On its own, the medical narrative isn't very inspiring. It's like the manual for my television remote: it is complicated, necessary, and potentially helpful, but it doesn't tell you anything about me. It doesn't tell you who I love, or what I like on my pancakes, or how I've lived with or made sense of suffering and illness.

In a 2009 TED Talk called "The Danger of a Single Story," Nigerian novelist Chimamanda Ngozi Adichie described how every life and every culture is the product of stories layered on stories like geological strata. Human beings are diminished, robbed of our variegated, imperfect, and beautiful humanity, when we are reduced to a single story—"cancer patient," for example.

When you hear that I am a cancer survivor, you might imagine that I am tragically heroic, battling the disease, just like everyone else who has cancer. I am neither tragic nor heroic; most people with cancer aren't, either. In fact, as you will see, the battle metaphor is a bit of tinfoil in my teeth. I am much more than my illness, and my experience of illness is far more complex than any single metaphor.

This is a book of stories I've been told and that I tell about my cancer. Some of them have advanced my healing and enriched my life. Others have flattened me and my humanity into something one-dimensional. This is not a book about the failures of the medical system, nor is it about practical solutions for fixing it. There are plenty of ideas elsewhere about that. It is a book about humanizing our experience and understanding of illness in general and of cancer in particular.

Part One:
2006–2008

A Scar Near My Temple

It was more than twenty years ago when I first felt a small lump beneath the skin on the left side of my head. I knew that it could be one of any number of benign and unremarkable bumps of human tissue. Nonetheless, my bowels turned to water, my heart raced, and my mind caterwauled sounds of panic. Images of my fatherless children filled me with terror and guilt. I leaned over the sink for a closer look in the bathroom mirror. I broke out in a sweat. I squeezed it between my thumb and forefinger. It was probably cancer, and I would soon be dead. In the passage of mere seconds, I grieved our children's weddings, grandchildren, growing old with Pearl. I told her about the lump, but not my fears. "No big deal," I lied.

Later that week, I saw my family physician. "It's probably nothing," I said, "but there's this little lump on my head."

"Let's have a look." He pushed and wiggled it, checking to see if it was attached to my skull. It was. "Yep, there's something there, but like you said, it's probably nothing. Still, we should get it checked out."

He referred me to a plastic surgeon in Thunder Bay, west of our home in the Northern Ontario town of Marathon. Arrangements were made for day surgery. I got up early one spring morning and drove the winding three hundred kilometres to the appointment. I lay on my side on the examination table. The surgeon froze my head around the lump and commenced carving. He stretched the incision open like the mouth of a trout and scraped the knob from my skull with a scalpel.

"Have you ever been hit here on the side of your head?" he asked.

"Probably, but not anything big, not that I can recall," I said.

"Huh, strange," he replied, still scraping away. The sound of scraping, amplified by my skull, was like a dog on a bone. "Strange," he repeated, "this looks like scar material." He waved a grisly chunk of tissue in front of me, then dropped it into a plastic vial. It would be sent to London, Ontario, for a biopsy. He stitched up the incision, then continued to muse, "It's like you've had a wound near your temple."

I'm a religious guy and a storyteller. You can't say things like "scar near your temple" and expect me to just take it literally. The metaphor instantly took up residence in my heart. I drank a plastic cup of apple juice, ate a couple of Peek Freans cookies, and then headed home. As I drove, the doctor's words tumbled over and over in my mind like small stones in a polisher. I said them out loud: "Looks like scar material near your temple." I wondered: have I been wounded near my temple, that sacred metaphorical place within each of us?

Years earlier, in theological college, our Pastoral Care and Counselling professor arrived one morning and told us that he had been at home in bed, felled by a prostate infection. He said he lay there considering this condition. "Can't pee. Can't piss. Pissed off. Am I pissed off?" he had asked himself. "Yes, I am pissed off." He got out of bed, came to the college, and confronted a faculty colleague with whom he was pissed off. "I feel much better now," he told us and proceeded with the class. We seminarians were gobsmacked by the professor's recounting of his literal application of mind-body theory.

I've been intrigued ever since by theories about the ways our physical bodies can manifest our psycho-emotional states. While I was in pastoral ministry, I frequently recommended *Love, Medicine and Miracles* by American author and physician Bernie Siegel to parishioners suffering with health issues. I remain skeptical of strictly literal, pissed-off-prostate conclusions, but I am convinced that the separation of the physical from the psycho-emotional is an arbitrary and artificial concept. At the very least, physical illness is an invitation to reflect on the state of our psychological, emotional, and spiritual well-being.

After that first lumpectomy, driving home along the north shore of Lake Superior, I reflected on the possible wounds inflicted on my temple, the sacred place within me. My childhood, by most standards, was a good one; my score on the Adverse Childhood Experience (ACE) scale would be pretty low. I come from a relatively loving, healthy family. We weren't perfect, but we did pretty well. Still, even in the best of circumstances, children absorb traumas into their fragile spirits. I did.

My father was an admired man of strong opinions and a powerful personality. Our young mother was often over-whelmed by the antics of her three sons. My brothers and I were spanked—mostly "when your father gets home"—with a wooden paddle adorned with the words "Board of Education." One of my brothers was deeply troubled. Today, he would be labelled ADHD or something like it. Back then he was just "bad" and in need of discipline. I both feared him and worried about the problems he created for himself.

His troubles followed him into his teens. On many nights, I fell asleep listening to my brother and my father hashing things out downstairs at the kitchen table. I envied and resented their troubled intimacy. I withdrew and kept my own troubles as far from home as possible. As I saw it, I was protecting my parents by keeping my heartaches to myself. I wanted their approval, their "Atta boy's," and organized my life accordingly.

Machismo and put-down humour ricocheted around our house like bouncing balls. If someone's feelings got hurt, we said, "Just kidding." We rationalized our jibes as signs of affection. Our capacity to give and take teasing only testified to our closeness. I did my best to play along, but I was emotionally thin-skinned and easily hurt by the taunting.

I was a sensitive boy, given to play and activities considered girlish in the 1960s: cooking, the arts, creating stories, candle-making, making believe. I had GI Joes like the other boys, but unlike the other boys, I sewed clothes for them. I was melancholic, a daydreamer. For a long time, I was overweight and ashamed of my body, my pleasures, my lack of masculinity. I cried tears of happiness and sadness too easily. I buried my precious inner life to avoid ridicule and retreated into an imaginary life in which I was brave and heroic.

As a teenager, I continued to be drawn to visual art and theatre. In a failed attempt to live up to my misguided ideas about what it was to be a man (and to impress girls), I played high school football—mostly from the bench.

My parents referred to me as "the disappearing child," because I developed an uncanny radar for looming family conflicts and vanished before they started. I am still pretty good at reading the emotional temperature of a room, even if I don't know what's causing it.

In the final semester of Grade 9, I scored D's in French and math. That summer, I ran away from home. I hitch-hiked north and west and then east to Ottawa. Ostensibly, I was fleeing my parents' insistence that I attend summer school. The truth is a paradox. I wanted to disappear, and I wanted to be seen. Like a child running to his room in tears, I wanted to be left alone and followed.

Salvation for me came in long, solitary, early-morning runs. My training partner was God. I ran, and we talked every morning for miles through the streets of Windsor, Ontario. I felt heard and sensed a tender voice of love speaking to me. I got stronger on those runs—physically, emotionally, socially, and spiritually. I began to discover my true self. Those runs launched me on a lifelong voyage.

So the answer to my surgeon's question was, yes—I had some childhood scars near my temple.

A little while later, the results of the biopsy came back: all clear. And I began paying attention to the scars near my inner temple.

I found a spiritual director. Rev. Dr. Nancy Lane was a guide and companion for more than fifteen years. Our monthly conversations took place by telephone because she lives in Elmira, New York. Our early conversations were about healing my "inner child" by unpacking those wounds near my temple.

The little girl from Robert Munsch's children's book "*Giant; or Waiting for the Thursday Boat*" started showing up in my dreams. Pearl and I were reading it to our kids at bedtime. In "Giant," God is illustrated as a small African-American girl.

In one of those dreams, this little brown girl-God took me by my hand and led me down the stairs to the basement of my unconscious. In another, I was in a barn shovelling out a stall knee-deep with manure, and she showed up to help. I recall another dream in which I was barrelling down a highway at the wheel of a massive transport truck. The little brown girl-God climbed up the front grill. She popped her head up over the hood of the truck, smiled at me, and shrugged her shoulders.

The question about scar tissue near my temple became an invitation to healing. I was awakened to previously unknown parts of myself. It led to greater inner peace. My spirituality deepened, and my understanding of God expanded. I learned about forgiving myself and others, not just for specific wrongdoings, but forgiveness in the sense of welcoming—loving, even—our flawed, imperfect, and beautiful humanity.

The lump on the left side of my head reoccurred in the ensuing years. It required increasingly invasive surgeries. One involved peeling my scalp back from my left ear to the crown of my skull and scraping the underside like a rabbit pelt. Another excised muscle from my jaw. The side of my head gradually caved in, crisscrossed with fibrous scars. "Not to worry," the doctors told me. "It's benign. It just a dirty tumour that sends out spores like a mushroom."

I was not cured by the story about scars near my temple, but there was tremendous healing in listening to the wisdom in it.

Treasure Hunting

"It is by going down into the abyss that we recover the treasures of life," said mythologist Joseph Campbell. One of the stories I tell about my cancer is that it is an unwelcome blessing. In spite of the suffering, I've found some treasure in it.

In August 2006, at Lakehead University in Thunder Bay, Ontario, I was installed as the 39th Moderator of The United Church of Canada. It was a grand affair—the pinnacle of my vocation as a minister. For three years, I would serve as the spiritual leader of the largest Protestant denomination in Canada. Friends from our church in Marathon joined Pearl and I on the stage. A thousand voices sang, "Everything before us, brought us to this moment, standing on the threshold of a brand new day." It felt as though I was exactly where that One Love called me to be. For me, there is no greater joy than that.

After the ceremony, after the handshaking and the hugs, after the photographs and a press scrum, Pearl and I walked across the university campus. The McIntyre River whispered below as we crossed the footbridge. The aurora borealis danced green in the dark sky above. We marvelled at this remarkable thing happening in our lives.

I was ready. I had earned three master's degrees, plus certifications as a spiritual director and as an expressive arts therapist. I was theologically liberal, scripturally intelligent, and spiritually grounded. I could chair contentious meetings in non-anxious ways. My heart was set on justice. I was an accomplished writer and a damn good preacher—if I say so myself. As the second youngest moderator in the history of our church, I brought vitality and vision for the future. I envisioned myself leading the church into a new reformation. I still had a good head of hair, both eyebrows, and not nearly enough humility.

Lying next to Pearl back in the university dorm room where we were billeted, I felt a new lump near my temple; a disappointing but relatively minor nuisance on such a fine night. After all, the doctors kept saying it was benign—just a dirty little tumour sending out its fungal spores. No big deal.

Relocated from Marathon to Toronto, where The United Church of Canada is headquartered, I met with a surgeon at Sunnybrook Hospital. He had reviewed the stains from all of my previous biopsies, and the one from the excision he had just performed. "Mr. Giuliano," he informed me, "your tumour has been misdiagnosed for years. It is in fact malignant." He said some other things. His lips moved, but the sound of blood storming in my ears drowned out his words. My self-perception and my confidence in God's call were shaken to the core. How could someone sick and weak lead the church? Would cancer treatments incapacitate me?

Against my own instincts, I began to learn how to lead from weakness and vulnerability. I travelled across Canada and around the world, speaking from my fragility rather than strength. Cancer and its treatment knocked me from the saddle of the great white stallion of certainty, youth, and vitality. I started to ride a humble, sometimes comic, donkey, like the one Jesus rode into Jerusalem to face the power and fury of the Roman Empire.

Leonard Cohen sang, "There is a crack in everything / That's how the light gets in." In weakness, I came to know the inner light of compassion, wonder, and beauty, of the sacredness and miracle of simply being alive. My physical senses intensified. The sound of bees, the slant of sunshine through a window, the weight of a warm blanket, the scent of soil brought tears, or laughter, or both.

This brush with my mortality felt like a call to spend my transitory life on worthy endeavours, and paradoxically, I found renewed pleasure in mundane daily activities—commuting, cooking, cleaning, small talk—and in the fraternity, the sorority, of waiting rooms. Even the meetings that had previously made me restless and impatient became conduits of the sacred. The cracks caused by cancer let light in.

The Apostle Paul's words recorded in his Second Letter to the Corinthians—"We have this treasure in earthen vessels"—became a touchstone. I came to realize that each of us, as individuals and as communities, has a magnificent divinity within. We carry this treasure around in the fragile clay pots of our bodies. When those pots, our bodies, are cracked, the light not only gets in, but it also gets out.

Gord Downie, the front man of the band The Tragically Hip, died last week. We knew it was coming. He was told a year and a half ago that he had an untreatable brain tumour. He dedicated his final months to music and to speaking out about the injustices inflicted on the First Peoples of Canada. Many Canadians heard for the first time about the violent truth of our national history because Downie used the platform of his looming death to talk about it. Last words have power because we save our breath for what matters most. Downie lived his final days from a place of inner light and the power of vulnerability.

American author, professor, and social worker Brené Brown writes and speaks about the power of vulnerability in her 2012 book, *Daring Greatly: How the Courage to Be Vulnerable Transforms the Way We Live, Love, Parent, and Lead:* "Vulnerability is the birthplace of love, belonging, joy, courage, empathy, and creativity. It is the source of hope, empathy, accountability, and authenticity. If we want greater clarity in our purpose or deeper and more meaningful spiritual lives, vulnerability is the path."

Following that path demanded that I lead from humility and authenticity rather than achievement, vitality, and strength. I came to recognize our church as vulnerable, too, called to live out our relationship with the Creator through present losses rather than past victories. Once upon a time we were a powerful and respected institution. We wielded social authority. We had the ear of the prime minister. Our sanctuaries were full. At the dawn of the twenty-first century, we were shrinking, losing our place of privilege in society. We were being called to a more humble, vulnerable, and unfamiliar way of living out our faith in the world.

I began to plumb my own frailty for wisdom and encouragement that might guide our diminished community. I dug for the treasure within the earthen vessel of our body politic, watching for the divine light our cracked institution was admitting and releasing. The Swiss psychoanalyst

Carl Jung often famously said that "the shadow is ninety percent pure gold." I was digging for gold in the shadows of this newfound vulnerability, in myself and in our church. I tried to reframe our story through the lens of my own story of vulnerability.

Be Not Afraid

I am back at the moderator's residence in Toronto after the meeting with my surgeon where he told me my tumour had been misdiagnosed for years as benign. I am trying to remember everything he told me. I think he said he would remove the latest lump and perform a biopsy to confirm his diagnosis. But I'm not sure.

I haven't called Pearl yet. I haven't told our children Jeremiah and Naomi, or my parents. I haven't called anyone or spoken to anyone because I am terrified. Repeating that word—*malignant*—would make it true, real. I am terrified that my fear will infect Pearl and the children like a virus. I am afraid that I will have to let go of the beautiful love we share. I am afraid of being deprived of weddings and grandchildren and growing old in love with Pearl. I am afraid of being sick and weak, when I need to be strong and healthy to lead the church. I am afraid of painful surgery and chemotherapy and radiation treatments. I am afraid that I will be too weak to suffer nobly. I am not afraid of death, what-ever mystery it holds. Right now, death feels like a welcome escape from fear. If it must come, let it come quickly.

"Don't be afraid" was my message to the delegates who elected me to lead their church. "We live too much out of fear," I told them. "Fear keeps us from risking the future." I now realize I had no idea what I was saying—no concept of the cost, the price.

"Don't be afraid." These are not new words, or even my own. They are the ancient words spoken first by an angel at the annunciation to Mary of her pregnancy and again outside the empty tomb on the first Easter. They are words spoken countless times in the gospel story, before and after and in between. When they are spoken, the one who hears is being called to something new and quite often terrifying.

In my terror, I am trying to persuade myself of three things:

- Fear, when it is our master, becomes our enemy. I need to listen to my fear without giving in to it. I need to speak to it gently and with love. I tell myself, "Of course you are afraid; and you are faithful, and you are not alone."

- Faith, not courage, is what I need right now. Faith means trusting my relationship with God—not that

God will fix me, but that wherever cancer takes me, whatever happens, God is there with me.

- I need to be courageous too. Courage is going ahead even when we are afraid, when our faith is fragile. The word "courage" comes from the French word *coeur*, meaning heart. So, to find my courage I must find my heart—I must find the centre of my life and passion.

Fear is always about the future. I don't fear the past or even the present. I am afraid of what lies ahead. In this moment, I am paralyzed by fear, preoccupied with the suffering that might come. I need to breathe, seek peace, and be at rest in this moment. I need to accept that this is difficult right now because I am overwhelmed by the demons of my imagination.

I am welcoming and soothing my fear, listening to it, and putting it in its rightful place. I will pick up the phone, dial our home number, and cry with Pearl. I will tell Jeremiah and Naomi. I will choose to trust that love is greater than my fear.

Welcoming the Wound

*I*t's been a week since the surgery to remove the tumour and to confirm that it is malignant. That was the sixth go at it, I think. I can't keep track. With each procedure I've gained some scar and lost a little bundle of nerves. About a quarter of my scalp is numb. My left eyebrow is immobile.

I accidentally saw the damage done to my face. I tried not to see it. I didn't want to see how I had once again been defaced. When I went to have some of the stitches removed, I saw my face flash in the mirror on the wall of the surgeon's office. This is what I saw: a hole on the left side of my forehead as big around as a Canadian two-dollar coin and as deep as a stack of four of them. The hole is rimmed by a crusty blood-black web of tiny stitches anchoring the scrim of skin grafted there from my thigh. A six-inch incision curves from the top of the hole down my temple below my ear.

I am not a vain person, but I am accustomed to the face I have. Had. I like to recognize myself when I look in the mirror. With age, it has undergone some gradual, natural changes: wrinkles, some droop in my eyelids, a wattle beneath my neck. They fall into the category of "normal." This new damage was something else entirely.

Having seen this new hole in my head, I began to gingerly care for it, dabbing Polysporin onto the crusty rim with my finger, replacing the blood-brown dressing with a clean one.

The perfect roundness of the hole and the elegant downward curving trail of scarred flesh had a graceful symmetry about them. Were it not on my face, I might have found the shape actually attractive. I began to doodle it, transforming it into a sunflower with ink and imagination. A man praying on his knees, or limping with a cane. A wriggling sperm. I thought about getting it tattooed. Pearl said it looked like a flower. I started to leave it exposed, to the air and onlookers.

The swelling has shrunk. The hole is now downsized to the size of a nickel and as deep as a stack of only three of them. I'm trying to be curious about the story my body is telling. Maybe it is a story that will help me to be a wiser and more compassionate leader.

I'm coming to see that it isn't enough to achieve that elusive and final stage of grieving: acceptance. I want to learn to welcome this wound and this scar. I want to find beauty in them. Allow them to guide me to a union with the Divine.

Nancy Lane, my spiritual director, sent me a prayer with which to start each day. It is a prayer about welcoming everything, even those aspects of me that I would prefer not to welcome:

Welcome, welcome, welcome.
I welcome everything that comes to me in this moment
because I know it is for my healing.
I welcome all thoughts, feelings, emotions, persons, situations,
and conditions.
I welcome my fear.
I let go of my desire for security.
I let go of my desire for approval.
I let go of my desire for control.
I let go of my desire to change my situation, condition, person,
or myself.
I open to the love and presence of God and the healing action
and grace within.

Stories of Blame and Battle

*T*here are stories people tell about illness that I have not found healing. You've likely heard them or even told them before. They are familiar stories, ones that are broadcast frequently in the public square of the town called Cancer. We keep telling them. As long as we don't examine them too closely or follow them to their logical conclusions, they bring a measure of comfort.

"God is teaching you a lesson, testing your faith, or punishing you for some sin of commission or omission." These narratives still have currency in the fundamentalist circles of most religious traditions. They continue to lurk in the collective unconscious of our culture. We say things like, "God doesn't give us anything we can't handle," or, "This is teaching you to rely on God." Even more insensitively, the self-righteous say, "If you have enough faith, God will cure you."

I don't think of cancer as an act of God so much as a natural disaster, like floods and forest fires. Shit happens.

Liberal religionists like me reject the notion that the Great Mystery engages in punitive or pedagogical edification by inflicting illness. The One Love does not permit Job-like suffering to test the steel in our faith-bone. Neo-atheists and the progressive faithful alike rightly consider such notions cruel and intellectually dissatisfying answers to suffering.

"Everything happens for a reason": I hear that one all the time these days. What I think people mean when they say it is, "It is possible that something good can come of this bad thing." I realize that people who've said this to me are trying to reassure and inspire me. But I want to punch them in the nose.

"You mean like the Holocaust?" I'm tempted to ask. "Did that happen for a reason? What about the little boy who drowned last month? What was the reason for that? What about famine? What about Becky, who hung herself last year? I imagine there was a reason for that. She had her reasons."

Instead, I smile weakly while chewing on my tongue and keeping my fists in my pockets. I say nothing, because in a small town you can't go around punching kind, well-intentioned people in the nose. Nonetheless, "Everything happens for a reason" is one of the cruellest, most insipid, emotionally stunted, uninformed things you can say to someone who has cancer. Please don't.

Here's another narrative popular among the righteous healthy and medical professionals: "If you eat nutritious food, exercise, don't smoke, drink alcohol in moderation, and practise mindfulness meditation, you will remain healthy until you die peacefully in your sleep at a ripe old age." It turns the ill person into both victim and perpetrator.

As with the Christian story of the man born blind, somebody must have sinned. Somebody didn't lose weight, go for a walk, or sign on to a carb-free diet. This version of the self-help narrative has had some critical passages ripped out: chapters about the design of buildings and off-gassing of construction materials; about environmental toxins, the stress of modern life, and childhood trauma; and about being dealt a bad genetic hand at the blackjack table of life. "Live healthy and you won't get sick" is a delusion that comforts the healthy and blames the ill. By blaming my cancer on my lifestyle, the cancer-free can continue imagining that it won't happen to them.

I was once a subscriber to the "live right, be healthy" narrative. After all, I cross-country ski and snowshoe. I run, mountain bike, and kayak. I eat healthy. I don't smoke. I enjoy an occasional glass of red wine, but I never drink to excess. I pray. I meditate. And *I got cancer*. The effrontery.

And then there's the most pervasive story of them all: "Fight!" "Battle!" And why not? In North America, this is the reflexive reaction to anything that frightens us: drugs, terrorism, poverty, sugary soft drinks, cellulite. We declare war. We are fighters, not victims!

How many obituaries begin, "After a long battle with cancer . . ."? Battle narratives end with victors and vanquished. If you live, you are a winner. If you die, you are a loser. Sorry, but when I die—and we all will die someday, let's not kid ourselves—I don't want to die a loser.

The battle narrative drags me back to sixth grade. I am trapped in a circle of bloodthirsty classmates, all shouting "Fight! Fight! Fight!" My nemesis, Dom DelBello, has somehow achieved the height, weight, and facial hair of a middle-aged man by the time he is twelve years old. I, on the other hand, am still a squishy four-foot-tall 150-pounder. The only fight I might win would be a war of words—which is likely why Dom wanted to beat me up in first place. I remember the overwhelming feelings of panic, certain defeat, confusion, and shame that preceded those fights. I remember the self-loathing that followed them.

"You gotta fight this! You're a fighter!" That's what people say about my cancer. "You can kick cancer's ass!" Like a coach in the boxing ring, they want me to keep swinging. Maybe sometimes I need that.

There are times, though, when I'd rather curl up in the arms of my lover than march into battle. Times when love would be the healing thing. The battle narrative has no room for my fear or weakness. It ridicules my weariness. It will not tolerate my sadness. Those are the feelings of coward.

"New research shows that at least 20 per cent of patients develop PTSD within six months of diagnosis—a rate similar to that of combat veterans," reported the *Globe and Mail* recently. If our only narrative is battle, it should not come as a surprise that cancer patients suffer the same psycho-emotional trauma as soldiers.

The battle narrative motivates physicians and patients alike to pursue futile and even harmful treatments rather than wave a white flag.

I'll call her Alice. She was in her late seventies and had cancer of the mouth and throat. Two surgeons and her oncologist had told her that they could do no more. Her cancer was rapidly spreading in her jaw and metastasizing to other organs. But Alice persisted until she found a surgeon willing to remove most of her lower jaw, even though he too told her it would not stop the cancer.

I visited her in hospital after the surgery. Her lower jaw was gone. Her dressings oozed. When I asked her how she was doing, she scrawled on piece of paper: "I'm a fighter!"

Alice lived a few more months in gruesome, drugged, and excruciating agony. Then she died. Her obituary announced that she had lost her battle with cancer.

The battle metaphor also makes me an enemy of myself, makes an enemy of the cells of my own body. So, illogically, I am fighting myself. Who else is there? Dom DelBello has left the playground. Cancer is not some external invading army. My cells have gone rogue, I'll grant you, but they are mine, they are part of me, part of my body. So how does one love one's body and at the same time declare war on it?

Again, I'm not saying that cancer is a good thing. I am not happy about it. I think, though, that healing—and with any luck, curing—requires complex diplomacy, negotiation, care, and love, not a grenade launcher.

The battle metaphor is a story about violence, not healing. Let's be honest: no geopolitical war has ever led to peace in the world. The war on terrorism we are currently fighting has only led to more fear and all manner of bad choices. It seems unlikely that doing battle will lead to peace or healing in me either.

Some of these stories—of blame and battle—may provide some consolation and encouragement for some people. If you understand your suffering as an act of God or solely the consequence of poor lifestyle choices, so be it. If the battle narrative consoles or inspires you, fine. I don't want to rob you of whatever comfort you find in them. They don't work for me. Letting them go has drawn me deeper into mystery and the unpredictability of life.

Darkness

Tonight I had a CT scan and an MRI at the Princess Margaret Hospital, which everyone tells me is the best cancer facility in Canada. My surgeon and oncologist are world-renowned. My CT was scheduled for 6:00 p.m. and the MRI for 11:00 p.m., but both were completed in a friendly "let's-move-it-along-and-please-don't-swallow" fashion by 8:30 p.m.

Now I'm down the street at the Second Cup rewarding my courage with a butterscotch nut tart and a decaf latte. The truth is, courage tonight came in the form of the two Ativan tablets that I put under my tongue to quell my claustrophobia before being stuffed into the MRI tunnel. MRIs still summon a childhood memory of a snow-tunnel cave-in. Now I've got the munchies.

Hot Latin music is playing loud. The coffee is good, even in a paper cup. My laptop keyboard is gooey with tart filling (apologies to the guys in IT). The baristas—one guy, one gal—are giggling about a good-looking boy who just left the shop smiling back at them over his shoulder. The city is alive and revelling in the warm spring night. Darkness is settling in like a friend. My folks are attending the opera tonight. We aren't generally an opera-attending clan. They are celebrating Dad's birthday and Mother's Day. Life is good. Life is very good.

These days I often hear my own words from church friends and strangers: "Don't be afraid!" When I first spoke them they seemed sublimely inspired. Now that I am really learning about fear, they seem so insubstantial.

Tonight, I am not afraid. Yes, there will be some more pain and facial disfigurement and loss of capacity ahead. The prognosis ain't pretty, but it is good. This cancer probably won't kill me.

My mantra continues to be "Trust." Trust that I am not alone. The hundreds of e-mails, cards, prayers, and stories of encouragement I receive lift my spirits and engage my curiosity. I wish I could respond personally to each and every message. And trust my relationship with the One Love, with the Great Mystery, with the Presence that I have known since I was a little boy.

I am learning to walk in the valley of shadows. I've lived most of my life in the light and on mountaintops. Now I'm digging for what can be mined from the soul in the dark. I have become a student of the paradoxical coexistence of joy and sorrow, of transformation and loss, of faith and fear. Who knows where it will lead? Tonight, like the warm dark night that pulses outside the coffee shop, it excites me.

Tonight, I feel strong in the Spirit. My heart soars with the possible blessings of this unwelcome, unlovely intrusion in my life. And I don't think that's just the Ativan talking. Like a spring bulb, or the roots of an apple tree before blossom, I sense something is stirring in the dark beneath the soil.

Tomorrow the surgeon will give me the low-down. Together we will decide what is next. For now there is sweetness in my mouth and an invitation to the dark night and the promise it holds.

The Tabernacle of God

*T*his morning, I took the subway to yet another pre-op appointment, this time at the Toronto General Hospital.

I spent the day rebelling against the dehumanizing nature of these clinics. Waited for the receptionist to look up from her screen, to make eye contact before I spoke. Made small talk with other anxious pre-op patients. Asked for, remembered, and used the name of each staff person I encountered.

Nancy from the lab took four vials of blood from my arm. She put stickers all over my body and wired me up for an EKG (which inexplicably stands for "echocardiogram." Why the K?) She apologized after ripping each of the stickers off the hairy bits of my body. *Rip.* "Sorry." *Rip.* "Sorry."

Angela put a cuff around my arm and measured my blood pressure. She counted how many times my heart beat in a minute. She recorded my weight and height. She quizzed me: Allergies? Alcohol? Recreational drugs? Smokes? "No, yes, not for a long time, and no." She described the day of surgery, and in more gruesome detail than I felt necessary, what would be done to my face.

I asked how long I might be in hospital (a week) and if I could pick the music that would play in the operating room during my surgery. I wanted Leonard Cohen (*Ten New Songs*), Van Morrison (*Avalon Sunset*), and the Blind Boys of Alabama (*Higher Ground*). Angela said to bring some CDs and see what the surgeons say. In heaven, God might pick the tune and harps the angels play. But in operating rooms, the surgeons are the gods of the iPod.

By the time the poking and prodding was finished, I was finished too. I needed a nap. It is exhausting to assert one's peculiar humanity in an environment reliant on uniformity, efficiency, and consent.

On the subway ride home, I half dozed and half read a chapter from teacher and theologian Marva J. Dawn's 2001 book, *Powers, Weakness, and the Tabernacling of God*. The chapter I was reading was about the Apostle Paul and his conviction (which I described earlier) that God dwells in his weakness. God defeats the powers and principalities of the world through our weakness, smallness, and vulnerability.

I get this idea, intellectually, theologically. I've preached it countless times. I've explained it, but I've mostly done so from a place of vitality and power. There on the subway, after a gruelling day of hosting my fears and my failing body, I wanted to "get it below the neck," wanted to know it in my guts. Could God be tabernacling in my brokenness?

I shut the book, marking my page with a finger, and set it down on my lap and closed my eyes. I prayed for help truly seeing God in weakness.

The subway train rolled to a stop. I opened my eyes just as the doors opened. A very small young man stood in the doorway—a "little person," someone with dwarfism. His right leg was casted from toes to knee, his spine canted to the left, and his fingers blunt. He looked to be fifteen or sixteen years old. He wore a backpack and a scuffed running shoe on the un-casted foot. His brown hair was slicked and parted with school-picture-day precision. Giant aviator sunglasses covered most of his face. Propelling himself with a crutch onto the car, the doors closed behind him.

There were several vacant seats between us, but without hesitation he bypassed them all and hopped up beside me. His shoulder pressed against my arm. He looked up at me and smiled. He held my image in the mirrored lenses of his aviators. His legs swung above the floor. At the very next stop he hopped down and exited the train. The familiar subway chimes announced the doors were closing, and he was gone. It was all so sudden. He was there and then he vanished.

Stunned, I rested in the assurance that the One Love, the One who makes a home in my broken body, a fragile vessel, had honoured me with a visit, allowed me a transitory glimpse of Presence, a comfort on this day of pre-op preparations. "So," I smiled and said to myself, "so that's what the tabernacle of God looks like on the Bloor subway line this afternoon."

Grace in the Valley of Shadows

On Monday, I was anaesthetized while James Taylor and Van Morrison played on Dr. Gilbert's iPod speakers. I had requested Leonard Cohen too, but he nixed Leonard—"a downer," he said. He counter-offered James Taylor, which was okay. You don't want your surgeon feeling down. Over the next nine hours, bone and skin were excavated from my head and repaved with bone from my scapula and flesh from my back. Blood vessels were plumbed into new connectors.

I awoke to Pearl's sympathetic smile and assurances that all had gone well. Distant lightning strikes and the rolling thunder of pain made me grateful for the clouds of opioid cotton upon which I floated.

The days immediately following surgery were fogged by pain and their passing confused by narcotics. On Tuesday, after what seemed like hours of drug-induced sleep, I consulted the wall clock to discover that only four minutes had passed.

Percocet also convinced my mind that the wall at the foot of the bed—upon which the clock was mounted—was actually the ceiling. Disturbingly, I was hanging from the ceiling. The curtain separating my bed from that of my neighbour was falling sideways. I swapped the Percs for Tylenol 3's and suffered a little more in the cause of sanity.

On Tuesday, my parents came to sit with my Pearl and me. I sweated and slept most of the time they were there. It was lovely, though, floating in and out of that safe harbour, carried on the calm waters of familial conversation. Mom brought lilies of the valley from her garden. "For the valley," she said. They'd been reading a blog I started called *Postcards from the Valley*.

On Wednesday, I swallowed the hairball of dread caught in my throat and gave a quick peek in the bathroom mirror. Picture a middle-aged man with a couple of pounds of his back-flesh sewn to his face. Nicely sewn, mind you. Not like it was done by a Cub Scout working on his first badge. John Merrick whispered in my mind, "I am not an elephant! *I am not an animal!* I am a human being!"

On Thursday, the Very Rev. Sang Chul Lee and his wife, Shin Jah Lee, came to visit. Sang Chul was the moderator of The United Church of Canada from 1988 to 1990. We prayed and laughed together like old friends, though we were meeting for the first time. In fact, we laughed so hard that Mrs. Lee covered her mouth and asked Pearl if this face-stretching hilarity might dislodge the stitches anchoring the fresh flesh to my head.

Sang Chul knows that the Great Mystery sometimes calls us to lead in ways we would rather not. He was elected moderator the year the United Church agreed that gay and lesbian people could be ordained and commissioned as ministers. Sang Chul spent most of his term calmly absorbing the wrath of homophobic members of our church. It was not how he had imagined his time in office, not what he had had in mind. I hadn't planned to lead from a hospital bed, not what I had had in mind. His visit helped me trust that there just might be treasure in this unwelcome blessing.

Pearl brought me a card the morning after I first spied my face in the mirror. On the inside she wrote out the lyrics to Libby Roderick's song, "How Could Anyone":

How could anyone ever tell you
You were anything less than beautiful?
How could anyone ever tell you
You were less than whole?
How could anyone fail to notice
That your loving is a miracle?
How deeply you're connected to my soul.

Happy tears escaped between my swollen eyelids. Love does that to you.

Everybody Hurts

A William Blake wrote so eloquently in his poem "Auguries of Innocence:"

> *It is right it should be so*
> *Man was made for Joy & Woe*
> *And when this we rightly know*
> *Thro the World we safely go*
> *Joy & Woe are woven fine*
> *A Clothing for the soul divine*

Suffering is part of life. There. I've said it. Suffering in general and illness in particular are as all-natural and organic as the yogurt at your health food store. We live in a culture beset with imperatives of success, fitness, perfection, longevity, and the pursuit of happiness. Acknowledging that suffering is part of life feels like screaming obscenities in church. Like banging garbage can lids together during the cool-down after yoga. But, as R.E.M. sang in the 1990s, "everybody cries / And everybody hurts sometimes."

In North America, one of the stories that shape our worldview is that suffering and illness are abnormal, that they are signs of failure. They are anomalies in a life that is intended to be one of continuous well-being and happiness. Like the life you see in beer commercials or holiday brochures. No wonder there is so much secrecy and shame about illness. People with cancer—people like me—are failing at the story of the good life. We contradict and offend the preferred narrative.

In her 1995 book *Little Pieces of Light*, author and "spiritual midwife" Joyce Rupp writes, "Darkness is a natural part of life but I have fought this reality for years. Darkness always seemed like a powerful intruder into my light-filled life . . . [W]hen the dark moments did come, I felt that something had gone terribly wrong with me." Isn't that the story we've all been told, that darkness—spiritual or physical suffering—means something is wrong with us?

Suffering, however, is part of life right from the get-go. I have witnessed the brutal miracle of new life on two occasions. It appears to hurt. A lot. Definitely for Mom, and probably for the baby. We are birthed into the world by both joy and suffering. They are constant companions.

From birth onward, suffering is woven with the threads of ecstasy and wonder. Knees get skinned. Sticks and stones and words keep breaking hearts and bones. From colds to cancers, there is illness. Aging naturally involves suffering. I'm fifty-seven years old, and as Leonard Cohen said, "I ache in the places where I used to play." Even the very best death brings with it a measure of unavoidable physical and emotional pain for the dying and for the living. Grief is the photo negative of love.

Suffering is part of the deal. Philosophers and theologians have long laboured over the question of *why*. Ancient religious stories about God's punishment, testing, or lesson-teaching attempted to provide an answer. Contemporary equivalents tend to blame the victim—poor diet, not enough exercise—or attribute it to some cosmic and unknowable greater purpose—"everything happens for a reason."

To my mind, suffering is connected to freedom. For freedom to be meaningful, it must include the possibility of both joy and woe woven fine. Suffering is a necessity of creaturely evolution, and of the advancement of the human spirit. Freedom, both the predictability and randomness of it, is extended to all organisms, from whales to the cancer cells that have made a home in my head.

I am more interested in the question of *how* to best live with cancer, than I am in *why* I have it. How can I redeem this experience of illness? How can I allow it to make me a better person? How can this reminder of mortality help me love life more, and live it more deeply?

In the Christian tradition, there is a story about Jesus walking with his disciples and passing a man who has been blind since birth. The disciples ask Jesus, "Rabbi, whose sin—this man's or his parents' sin—caused this man to be born blind?"

Jesus' contemporaries believed that all suffering was caused by the sins of those who suffer, or the sins of their ancestors. The disciples were merely reflecting the culturally accepted answer to the question of *why*. Either the blind man (presumably in utero) or his parents had sinned. The list of sins was long. It included everything from the touching of a dead person to eating shrimp to blending fabrics and working on the Sabbath.

But listen to Jesus' reply: "Neither this man nor his parents sinned; he was born blind so that God's works might be revealed in him." Jesus changes the question from *who sinned* to *who will be revealed.* Who will be seen? (Note the irony: *they're talking about a blind man.* Get it? Never mind.)

So I wonder, *who* is my cancer revealing? Is my suffering glorifying—metaphorically speaking—God or the Devil? In other words, does my cancer amplify love or hate in the world? Am I becoming more compassionate toward the suffering of others because of it? Am I more awake to the miracle of life, having been reminded of its fleeting nature? Or am I becoming bitter, fearful, and more careful or closed off to the world?

As I write, Hurricane Harvey is wreaking havoc in Houston. Even more devastating rains are flooding parts of India, Bangladesh, and Nepal. These natural disasters, like all suffering, expose the best and worst in humanity. On one hand, looters are fleeing with televisions. On the other, people form themselves into human chains through raging waters to rescue strangers. Retailers price-gouge the desperate while neighbours paddle flooded streets in canoes to ferry the stranded to safety. A news story last night showed a woman going door to door, offering to do laundry for those whose homes have been ravaged. Humanity, at its best and its worst.

Why the hurricane, *why* the flooding are complex questions, and to a degree unanswerable: climate change, natural historic weather patterns, poor city planning, poverty, greed—the list is long. *Who* these natural disasters serve, to my mind, is a better question. Our response to suffering is more tangible and life-changing. One of the glories of freedom is that we have the capacity to choose between the best and the worst of our nature. At our best, we ask not *why* we are suffering, but *who* will it serve? What is it reveal-ing about us as human beings, about me?

Cancer has deepened my love, goodness, creativity, and generosity of spirit. At times it has also revealed less noble aspects of my character—my capacity for self-absorption, unkindness, and self-pity. I'll leave the question of *why* I have cancer to the philosophers and theologians. I want my illness to increase my capacity to live a more fully human, more awake, life. I want it to mean something.

I am not saying that suffering is good or desirable. I am not glad I've had cancer. But I want to experience the col-lateral beauty that sometimes accompanies suffering. That's one of the healing stories I tell myself about illness.

Paring Down

I've been paring down to the essentials.

I go to radiation treatments: a daily, grinding ritual of exhaustion.

I eat, even though everything tastes like bad peaches. You know the ones—they're round and firm and fuzzy in the store, but in your mouth they are dry and pulpy, the flavour of dust. Everything tastes like that to me. Good food these days is whatever doesn't cause me to gag.

I pray. However, the pillow set before the coffee table and the candle for the purpose of prayer is more often a place to lay my head than it is to sit upon in contemplation. I listen to Leonard Cohen's *Ten New Songs*. Lyrics like, "I am not the one who loves / It's love that seizes me / When hatred with his package comes / You forbid delivery." And, "As someone long prepared for this to happen / Go firmly to the window, drink it in." These words fill me with an unnameable emotion that can only be said with tears.

I go into the office, more for companionship than the accomplishment of work. They found a couch for me. I stretch out on it and return phone calls, glad for the human contact. I send a few e-mails. I nap beneath a flannel quilt sent to me in the mail by dear friends in Marathon.

On the way to radiation, I stop to sit on the concrete wall at the Queen's Park subway station, where I share some coins and friendly chat with Rick, who panhandles there. Last week, he noticed my hair falling out. He rummaged in his bundle, pulled out an electric razor, and gave it to me. "I've got two," he said while scratching the tangle of his long beard. We laughed until my eyes filled with tears. When I got up to go, Rick patted my shoulder and said, "Have good day."

I stay connected with Pearl across the miles by telephone. Sometimes I call Jeremiah and Naomi, but they're both away at school, and I don't want to worry them. If I have sufficient energy left, I call a friend. Most days I don't.

I am asleep most nights before 9:00 p.m., but it doesn't touch my heavy weariness. I wake up tired. I brush clumps of hair from my pillow. At night I sweep them out of the shower with a broom.

When you are sick, you have to practise an economy of energy. You have to decide what is essential to life and let everything else go. Even lovely, important, fun, or urgent things. It's hard to let go, but hanging on drains precious energy. Contemplating death—your own, or that of someone you hold dear—unveils a remarkable clarity. You wonder how on earth you spent so much time worrying about things that matter so very little.

These days, my pared-down life includes these essentials: kindness, generosity, forgiveness, and simplicity. I cannot afford to be anxious about things that hold no value in the economy of simplicity. Most people who brush up against their own mortality unearth the treasure of that truth.

Singing in a Strange Land

I would like to be able to say something encouraging, something about encountering the Holy One in the valley of shadows. Something about how, in the midst of the difficult week past, I sensed the presence of God nearby. I can't. If there is treasure, it remains hidden, buried.

I get up at 6:30 a.m., drink a coffee, and eat some cereal, hoping it will settle my stomach and the floogie feeling in my head. I take the subway downtown to the Princess Margaret Hospital. I am stubborn and take the stairs rather than the escalators. My muscles are atrophying. I rode my bike downtown for treatments on Monday and Tuesday, which raised questions around the office about my sanity. By Wednesday, I was too weak to ride. Thursday, I took the escalators. I was done for the week.

At the Princess Margaret, Lenny or Michelle or one of the other impossibly young radiation therapists calls my name. I remove my shirt and put on a gown that is immediately lowered to my waist as soon as I lie down. They ask me my birth date to confirm it's really me. I answer and say, "Be sure to send me a card." They smile, even though all the mirth has gone out of me.

A plastic mesh mask covers me chest to crown and bolts my head in place. It flattens my nose and presses against my throat. The eyes and mouth have been trimmed out of it in deference to claustrophobia. The technicians repeat numbers and calibrations to one another. I don't know what they mean. I don't care what they mean.

Then, in a bizarre coupling of high- and low-tech, my eyelid is taped up into the "target area" on my brow. The technicians instruct me to look down toward my toes on their cue. Failing to do so could leave me blind. Try it sometime. Tape your eyelid to your forehead. Then hold a downward gaze for two or three minutes, with the full knowledge that if you look up you might never see again.

The technicians are huddled in a lead bunker. I relax, slowing my heart and breathing. I visualize golden light flowing to my muscles and inner organs. Then a tinny voice from a speaker on the wall says, "Okay, look down." My toes curl reflexively, and I point my eyes in their direction. The multimillion-dollar machine hums to life, and my forehead is blasted with radioactivity. A metallic, acrid smell fills the air. We do this five times, five days a week.

The mask leaves my face waffled. The burned patch reddens and browns like meat on a spit a little bit more each day.

I feel increasingly lousy in nondescript ways. "Woozy" is the best word I can come up with. Nauseated, weak, tired, weird. By Friday night, I am a train wreck.

Tonight, I am telling myself two things. The first thing is that I am too weak to experience the Light. My incapacity to feel it, however, does not mean that the Light—God—is more or less close to me. The nearness of the Great Mystery is not limited by my capacity to recognize Her holy presence.

The second thing I am telling myself is that this is foreign territory. I have not been in this land of illness or fragility before. I am learning to pray in a new way, on difficult terrain. It is not easy to sing the Lord's song in a strange land, says the Psalmist, not easy to sing in a land to which one has been carried off in captivity (Psalm 137).

After I posted a blog about this, two profoundly encouraging pastoral responses showed up in the comments box. Rather than try to jolly me, the first affirmed my emotional state. It simply said, "I hate fucking cancer."

The second comment reminded me of the importance of community. "We'll sing the Lord's song for you," wrote the reader, "until you can sing it again."

Hope Changes Everything

*L*ittle children toss and turn in their beds. "How many sleeps?" they ask, until Christmas or their birthdays. Prisoners toss and turn on their narrow beds and count "get-ups" until the day of their release. I'm counting both sleeps and get-ups until Wednesday, when nine long weeks of radiation treatments come to an end, and I am set free to recover from what is meant to cure me. Thursday feels sweet on the tongue because that is when I'll fly away, oh glory, home to Marathon.

Medically speaking, I am at my most depleted state. My head is saturated with the maximum allowable levels of radiation. My tongue is a dry brick. Food tastes of wood and tinfoil. My left ear is burned to the consistency of beef jerky; I imagine dogs slathering with Pavlovian longing when I pass by them. The eye adjacent to the chewy ear is pink and swollen, my vision fuzzy. My hair is a distant and wispy memory. And, I'm beginning to feel great—emotionally and even physically.

What has changed is that the object of my hope is near. The promise of what lies ahead is already transforming the present. I am experiencing what scholars of biblical Greek call the "aorist tense": something that is "already and not yet." That is the nature of the gospel promise: what we hope for, dream of, and anticipate with certainty reaches back toward us from the future to transform the present.

My cancer pales in comparison to the great sufferings and hopes of this world. But today, I better understand how critical hope is for the transformation of the world.

Hope radically changes not only the future, but also the present. It changes nothing, and it changes everything. Five more sleeps and four more get-ups, and I am feeling better than I should after being irradiated for nine weeks.

It's a cliché, and like all clichés it contains a kernel of truth. We say, "Where there is life there is hope." It is also true that, "Where there is hope there is life."

Unrecognizable

$\mathcal{I}$ am back home in Marathon. Yesterday, I dropped by to say hello to Kim Stadey, a member of our church, at her "Styles for You" salon. I stepped through the door out of the rain, and she didn't recognize me. She smiled at me from behind the counter the way we smile at strangers: friendly, curious, careful. I doffed the ball cap from my bald head and demanded a trim. Then she recognized me. My voice, I think, was the giveaway.

People don't recognize me these days, even though they've known me for years. They know my voice, of course. They've listened to it in worship, at funerals, weddings, and community meetings, and while I hold court in the coffee shop. My face, however, is a puzzle to them.

I look different. My head is as bald as a baby's. My left eye is wonky. There is a pound of my back-flesh grafted to my face. I am different inside. Maybe they see that too: in my posture, in my stride. How I move feels different to me.

I'm not surprised that I'm unrecognizable, even to my dear friends and neighbours. It's disconcerting for them and for me. I hardly recognize myself when I look in the mirror.

Cosmetic procedures could make the new me look more like the old me. The plastic surgeon suggested implanting powerful "earth" magnets under my scalp to tether a toupee to the hairless side of my head. "You can swim with it," he assured me, "or hang upside down." I'm not getting the magnets but am enjoying describing them to friends. The telling usually includes a dramatization of me passing through airport security.

Hair plugs could be harvested from the other side of my head and planted on the bald side. I am picturing Naomi's childhood dolls with their hair-plug heads.

On my dresser, there's an unused referral slip to an eyebrow replacement specialist. Wiry hairs from one eyebrow or the back of my head could be transplanted to where the other used to be. Getting them at the right angle is a highly technical skill. Or I could have an eyebrow tattooed on. I think I'll go brow-less.

Dr. Gilbert wants to reduce the thickness of the flesh-flap. It kind of puffs out still. Jeremiah thinks I should get it done. "You have to talk in public a lot," he reasons. "You don't want to be up there talking about important stuff and meanwhile everyone is wondering, 'What's that thing on his head?'"

When asked about getting some cosmetic work done, I laugh and say, "Pearl still thinks I'm good-lookin', and that's all that matters to me." Which is true.

I am not the same person I was when I entered the valley of unwelcome blessings. Should my outer appearance not reflect my inner change? It feels wrong to camouflage the modifications writ large on my face; they tell a story. It feels wrong to be ashamed of the rearrangement underway in my life.

Miracle Cures

*Y*esterday afternoon, Jeremiah and I were in the basement repairing the foosball table. He and some friends took it in the back of a pickup truck to a party. The truck got stuck in the snow. One thing led to another, and one of the foosball table's legs broke off. He picked up bolts and advice at the hardware store and drilled out the stripped holes. We were in the process of gluing and screwing the broken piece back in place. I was enjoying the work, and even more so the time spent with our son.

Upstairs, the telephone rang. Pearl answered. The call was for me.

I picked up the receiver and said hello. The voice on the other end spoke with rapid familiarity. "Hi, David, do you have a few moments to talk?"

The needle on my telemarketer radar quivered. "I'm kind of in the middle of something right now. Can I ask what you're calling about?"

The caller ignored my question. "When would be a good time to call back?" The needle bounced into the yellow zone.

"How 'bout you tell me what you're calling about," I counter-offered, "and I'll let you know if there is a good time to call back."

"Well, I'm calling about your cancer . . ."

I don't even know this person's name, and he is calling me about my cancer?

He speaks quickly, telling me he has access to a cancer cure researched for a decade at McGill University in Montreal. It was endorsed by twenty research physicians. Maybe it was twenty years and ten research physicians. I was tuning out. There was something about a conspiracy by big pharma to keep the research from getting out to the public.

"I'm happy with the treatment I'm getting, thanks," I replied, trying to politely end the conversation.

He ploughed ahead as though I hadn't spoken. "These supplements—"

"I'm not looking for an alternative treatment," I interrupted. "I don't want to be rude, but I'm going to hang up now." And then I hung up. Firmly. Just shy of slamming the phone down.

Why was I so bugged about a guy calling who claimed he could save my life? How was it different than me offering to help Jeremiah fix his foosball table? (Other than the obvious differences between my head and a foosball table.)

For one thing, I don't know this man, and he doesn't know me. Relationship: that's the biggest difference. He spoke as though we had met, but didn't tell me his name. He doesn't know anything about me or my cancer. Apparently, the supplements he's hawking work on *all* cancers. He would have no way of knowing the rare sarcoma that went forth and multiplied on my left temple. *I* can't even remember the name.

I was bugged about a stranger breaking and entering our home, my life. I was bugged by his phony intimacy. I was bugged that he interrupted my time with our son. I was bugged by his dismissal and derision of the treatments and physicians I was choosing.

Where did he get my home number? Where was he calling from? I pictured other people, more desperate and frightened than me, being preyed upon by purveyors of "miracle" cures.

I've put my story of cancer out there on my blog, so I guess it's inevitable that I'll receive some unusual and well-meaning, if misguided, offers of help. Still . . .

The call bugged me for the same reasons that evangelical door-knockers bug me. They don't know me, but are convinced that my current state of eternal damnation can only be rectified by what they offer. My story doesn't matter. Not even my name. All that matters is the damnation story they want to tell.

I want to tell people about Jesus. But before the telling comes listening, comes learning—stories and names. I must first respect what other people love, what they are in the middle of doing, and what path of healing they are already following.

Healing and Curing

Sometime back in the early 1990s, I read an article in the *Utne Reader* called "How AIDS Saved My Life." It was written in an era of widespread homophobia and alarm about the transmission of HIV and AIDS. It told a courageous story.

The author wrote that prior to being diagnosed with AIDS, he, like most gay men of his generation, led two lives—a secret life and a public life. In his public life, the author pretended to be heterosexual. He had legitimate fears about being rejected by his family, colleagues, and neighbours. So he hid his true self from all but his closest gay friends. His soul was split between his true self and his false self. He was a broken and divided person.

He was diagnosed with HIV and later began to suffer the symptoms of AIDS. His illness inevitably revealed his hidden self to others. He began to live one undivided, true life. What was broken began to heal. What was divided came together. He reconnected with his parents and siblings. They struggled with his homosexuality but loved him in his need and vulnerability. He came out to his co-workers. Some of them had already figured out that he was gay and had collaborated in his deceit. Not all of them were willing to accept him and remain in his life. Some were afraid of contracting HIV.

As his physical health diminished, his wholeness as a person expanded. His relationships within his family deepened. He became more compassionate and accepting of his true self. "AIDS," he wrote, "saved my life."

An editor's note at the end of the article informed readers that the author had died prior to publication. AIDS saved his life, and it killed him. He was healed, but he was not cured.

That's how I remember his story, thirty years later. It is a story, I think, about the difference between healing and cure. We tend to use those words—"heal" and "cure"—interchangeably. To my mind, they are not synonymous. I find it helpful to distinguish between them when I talk about my cancer, and about what it means for me to experience healing or be cured.

A cure refers to the relief of the symptoms of a disease or condition. It is a matter of clinical pathology. You have a headache, and you take an Aspirin. The headache goes away; it is cured. You have a malignant tumour and treat it with radiation, chemotherapy, or surgery. If it goes away, you are cured. It is a binary word: you are cured, or you are not cured. It goes away, or it doesn't.

I think of healing as something more multidimensional, holistic, and all-encompassing. Healing means being restored to or discovering wholeness. It includes every aspect of the person—physical, psychological, relational, ethical, spiritual. Unlike a cure, healing is an ongoing, life-long labour. We are never completely healed. We are never "all better." We live our lives moving towards, and at times away from, healing.

After surgery and nine weeks of radiation therapy, my oncologist read the post-treatment MRI on the computer screen in the examining room. He thumbed and poked the edge of the surgical flap on my forehead. Then he crossed his fingers and drew a quick breath through his teeth, and in his lovely Irish brogue he said, "I think we've got it." I was—fingers crossed—cured of cancer. Given previous multiple recurrences, I was somewhat skeptical, but I also hoped that the more aggressive approach taken this time would be the charm.

Along the way, there has been healing. The recurring reminder of my mortality has been a clarion call to love life while it lasts. Not that it has made me a saint or a sage. I am still an imperfect, fragile, and fallible human being. I am not healed, but I am healing. I am becoming a more self-accepting, forgiving, gentle person. My relationships are deepening. I am more profoundly aware of the beauty and miracle of life. My capacity for loving and being loved has grown. I laugh more and am more accepting of my propensity to tears. I am less willing to squander what poet Mary Oliver calls my "one wild and precious life."

Cures and healing are intimately woven together. One, however, can occur without the other. We can be cured and remain unchanged, asleep to life and clinging to fear. In my case, I cannot say with any certainty that I have been cured, but I am healing. That's a story I am still learning.

Un-sudden Change

"*W*e all dream of having some kind of spectacular conversion," writes philosopher, theologian, and humanitarian Jean Vanier in *Befriending the Stranger*, "in which everything in our lives suddenly changes completely . . . and forever."

It's been a frustrating week at home. Things are not changing at a spectacular pace. Oh, there have been wonderful things about it—sleeping in my own bed, spooning with my beloved. On Sunday, we hosted a send-off feast in our backyard for all the young people heading off to school and new adventures. I got to watch our twenty-year-old son, Jeremiah, perform two of his songs at the Pic River First Nation Idol contest. Naomi and I drove over to Schreiber so she could take her driving test. She passed. I've managed a couple of short walks.

I still feel tired and weak most of the time. My taste buds have not re-sprouted. My jaw aches and is as stiff as an old leather boot. My eye is infected. My hair will never grow back. They told me it takes time to recover after radiation treatments. I was counting on them being wrong.

I want to be healed instantly like Jesus healed the ten lepers. The blind. The lame. Van Morrison's lyrics "Give me my rapture *today*..." keeps looping in my brain. I am impatient with being a patient. I want to be transformed now—this instant, dammit—like Paul on the road to Damascus. Wham! The road to Damascus, it turns out, is now longer than it used to be.

There were days in this valley carved by cancer when I thought, *This changes everything. I'll never be the same.* That's what I thought. I now see that I am changed, and I am not changed. I am still the same old imperfect, impatient human creature I've always been.

Sure, I see colours more intensely, appreciate stillness more fully, savour touch more freely. My love for my family and friends has grown. So has the pleasure I take in them. Even scarred, disfigured, and bald, I can see myself as beautiful.

And . . . I am impatient, critical, irritated, and distracted by the small details of life. I am healed and not healed, changed and not changed, by the unwelcome blessing of darkness.

"Jesus wants us to place at his feet all that we are carrying in our hearts," continues Vanier, "and to rest quietly with him; trusting that we are gradually growing in his love." The Christ longs for union. Ideas about "all-better-ness" can get in the way of union. Ideals of perfection distract us from it. When we love and welcome the, at times, unlovely crucified Christ, we can welcome our own, at times, unlovely crucifixions. The Christ of the gospels is not a Superman of triumph and victory, but rather the one who accepts the cross with all who suffer.

Part of healing is to lovingly welcome the imperfections and wounds that persist in us. Our imperfection is often the pathway God follows into our hearts. I wish I could learn to do that faster.

Unremarkable

*A*med student did the initial post-radiation examination for Dr. O'Sullivan, my oncologist. She poked and prodded. She asked how I was feeling and wrote down what I said. She seemed very nervous. I felt like saying, "Relax, you're not the one with cancer!" But I didn't think it would help.

Dr. O'Sullivan joined us in the examination room. The student gave him the update. She began by saying "This patient is unremarkable." Shocked, I looked at Dr. O., who smiled and winked. Apparently, being unremarkable is—medically speaking—a good thing.

Nothing showed up on the chest X-ray. A recent MRI scan revealed no signs of cancer. I've been feeling good and happy to be back out on the ski trails.

Dr. O'Sullivan looked me over. He squeezed and pushed at the side of my head. He slid his hands over my bald scalp in search of lumps, commenting in his hint-of-Irish accent, "I see you've got it right down to the wood."

That's when he crossed his fingers, sucked air through his teeth, smiled a grimacing sort of smile and said, "I think, well you can't ever, well, say for sure, especially with these rare types of cancer, but I think we've got it."

He's a lovely man and delivered some darn good news— the best one is likely to get from an oncologist. He and my surgeon have been a creative and accommodating team. There is the added pleasure of their names being Gilbert and O'Sullivan. I hope that someday together they will pen "The Pirates of Princess Margaret."

I am beginning to feel less frail and more and more "unremarkable." My own little energy crisis persists, but my smouldering coals of vitality are being fanned back to life. My playful self is picking itself up off the floor. I feel less and less like a bunch of bones in a flesh-bag.

Not that I want to leave the gifts of the valley of shadows behind. Frailty and vulnerability brought with it tenderness and a new kind of access to my inner life. It taught me to move more slowly, with greater intention and awareness. Priorities became clear. I couldn't waste precious energy on unimportant things. Each day was a blessing and a gift. Gratitude flowed naturally in me.

Walking back up University Avenue to College Street, I found myself smiling. I really am quite remarkable. So too are Dr.'s Gilbert and O'Sullivan. So too is the medical student who pronounced me unremarkable. I hope she knows just how remarkable she and every patient she examines is. Same with the cashier at the Tim Hortons in the hospital lobby. I want to shout to the people brushing up against me on the sidewalk, "Do you have any idea just how remarkable you are!" Do you? How remarkable is this life? When my eyes accidentally meet those of a stranger, I try to convey with a smile, "I see you, and I see that you are remarkable."

Part Two:
2015–2017

Involuntary Pilgrim

*A*s cancer has recurred in my life, another story has become important to me. It is a story about illness as an involuntary pilgrimage. It is the story of my Camino de Cancer.

Mecca, Machu Picchu, Lourdes, and Graceland are all well-known pilgrimage destinations. Perhaps the most familiar is the Camino de Santiago. It begins in France, and by various routes, leads to the Cathedral of Santiago de Compostela in northwestern Spain, where the bones of Saint James are reputed to be buried. People walk it for all sorts of reasons. Some people go for the exercise and physical challenge. Others go looking for community among fellow travellers. Still others seek healing, wisdom, or spiritual meaning. *Camino de* means simply "the way" or "the road."

Not all pilgrimages are geographical. Some are made invisibly, inwardly—journeys of the soul.

Matthew Fox, a former Dominican priest and founder of the Fox Institute for Creation Spirituality, described four paths or ways of the spiritual journey. The *Via Positiva* is the way of ecstasy, joy, eroticism, and delight. The *Via Creativa* is the way of creativity and co-creation and includes, for example, the encounter with the Holy through the practice or pleasure taken in the arts. The *Via Transformativa* is the way of struggle for justice, healing and compassion. By participating in changing the world, we are ourselves transformed. The fourth, the *Via Negativa* is a way of darkness, chaos, suffering, silence, and letting go and letting be. The *Via Negativa* is rarely chosen or even welcome. It comes upon us, abducts us, and we choose to walk and listen— or not.

I have walked all four of these paths in my spiritual journey. Over the past twenty years, I have at times found myself walking the inward way of the *Via Negativa*. I have tried to redeem the malignant presence of cancer by walking with it. On my Camino de Cancer, the disease has been the source of suffering and a harsh teacher of wisdom. It has been unwelcome, and it has been a blessing. Periodically, it comes banging on the door of my soul like a drunk and hostile stranger.

Eli Comes Calling

Pearl and I were still in our pyjamas, eating breakfast at home in Marathon when Eli Orrantia tapped on the kitchen window. Luna, his malamute, stood beside him on the deck.

The northern summer was drawing to a close, but the sun was still warm that morning. Eli and I sat side by side in the old Adirondack chairs, facing the trees. Dew turned to vapour above the strawberry patch. The spruce trees stood motionless, undisturbed by the light breeze. Luna lay down, planting her chin on my moccasin.

Eli is a dear friend. He is also my doctor. "I've got my doctor hat on this morning," he said.

"Okay," I replied.

"The other night, I was looking at that lump on your head," he told me. "I don't like the look of it."

We had all been at a wedding on Saturday. Everyone at our table told uproarious stories about their weddings and

85

how they had met one another. We drank wine, danced, and laughed our faces red.

"Me neither," I said, "but they say it's just scarring, or a nerve bundle, or something. The MRIs all come back clear."

"I don't believe the MRI," Eli countered.

The lump was above my left eye and to the right of my temple, which is already disfigured by my previous surgeries. I pressed on it with the heel of my hand. It felt like a budding horn beneath the skin. Given the choice between Eli's judgment and that of a million-dollar magnetic resonance imaging machine, I'd choose his. Hands down. Besides, his doubts only confirmed my own misgivings.

Stoicism is my usual first response—my go-to in fearful times. Denial and bargaining aren't my way. Instead, I surrender. That's life. What're you gonna do? I do not offer this observation as prescriptive or with apology. It is just what I do.

I sighed. "Okay. What now?"

"I'd like you to go back down to the Princess Margaret. See the oncologist and the surgeon again. Check it out. Just to be sure." *Just to be sure*, but he knows already. So do I.

We sat on my deck silently, breathing in the scent of strawberries, cedar, and spruce trees. The pungent smell of compost lifted on a warm huff of air. In the distance, a lawnmower barked to life.

Eli rested his hand on my forearm. "I'd just feel better if we checked it out."

"Well, okay," I said, "if it'll make *you* feel better." We laughed.

I don't recall Eli and Luna leaving, whether they took the path through the woods or went out front to the street. My head was elsewhere. I took a deep lungful of air, blew it out, and went inside to tell Pearl.

That's how it begins. One moment, it's breakfast, sunshine, and strawberries, and the next, *Via Negativa* comes knocking on the door of your soul. It sneaks in like a thief at night. No need to go looking for it; it finds us.

Embarking on this involuntary pilgrimage requires tying up our boots and slinging on a backpack containing only the bare essentials. We can't bring along all of the puny concerns that weigh down our normal day. We have to leave behind our shame about being weak and our fears of disability, in a world that idolizes strength, certainty, and independence. Our voice might break, but we need to share the bad news with those we trust to walk beside us. Allow ourselves to again be broken open to suffering and grace and blessing, to all of the beauty we've been overlooking. Cry joy over the miracle of being alive—the way we would every day, if we were paying attention.

Raphael's Promise

In Toronto, my old pals Dr. O'Sullivan and Dr. Gilbert and an MRI all agree with Eli's and my own suspicions. It's back. Surgery is scheduled for October. I slept on the flight home, and woke up remembering a phone call from my father.

The call came in 2007, while I was undergoing radiation treatments during my last bout with cancer. Dad, who's gone now, wanted to visit me. He would drive down from Owen Sound, Ontario, where he and my mom lived.

I told him not to come. "I am too sick," I said.

I have a high pain threshold and an above-average capacity for suffering, but I am private about it. I cope by going inside myself. When I'm sick, I lack the energy to host the questions and the anxieties of those who love me.

"I'll bring some food," he persisted, "We'll have lunch."

"Don't, Dad, please. Everything tastes like tinfoil. I can't keep anything down. The smells. And I'm just too tired to visit."

"You want comic books?" When my brothers and I were sick as kids, my father brought us ginger ale and *Archie* or *MAD* comics. I laughed in that tender way that catches in your throat and causes your eyes to sting. I was now forty-eight and a father myself. I've been known to bring comics and ginger ale to my own adult children.

"Dad, I'm just too tired to visit," I said again.

"Okay, we'll nap."

He came and we napped. My father dozed in a recliner, and I slept on a sofa, beneath a blanket despite the summer heat. Sunlight bathed the living room, illuminating our resting bodies.

My father's breathing changed. He was awake. He said, "I talked with Raphael. That's why I had to come today."

Raphael Giuliano, my great-grandfather, was a peasant from Naples, Italy, who immigrated to America. He was a widower and an irresponsible father. Soon after landing in New York City, Raphael married an opera singer and abandoned his six kids to the streets of Brooklyn. My grandfather was eleven years old when he last saw his father. So my father never met his no-good *Nonno*, Raphael.

"I have been praying to Raphael," my father said. "That's what I came to tell you."

"Thanks," I said, chastened.

"He came to me. Raphael."

I imagined Raphael, appearing to my father: smoking, wearing an undersized, threadbare suit, and a battered hat tipped rakishly on his head.

"I told him," my father continued, "'Raphael, you were a lousy father. You abandoned my father. He suffered a lot because of it. So did I.'" I could hear him swallow across the room. Our gazes were still fixed on the ceiling. "I told him that I was going to finally forgive him for all the pain he caused. Then I asked him to hear a father's plea for his son." My father paused. "Raphael promised to look out for you."

Looking up at the clear blue sky through the condo window, I watched a jet descend toward the Toronto airport. I whispered, "Thank you," and added, "Raphael, one of the archangels."

"Raphael means 'God heals,'" my father said. "So, we will be okay."

It was after he had gone—after we had embraced and kissed at the door, and I had laid back down on the sofa—that it occurred to me: He said *we*, not *you*, will be okay. *We* will be okay. We both would be okay.

My father has since joined his father and grandfather in the mystery of life beyond life.

My thoughts returned to the present. Through the window of the plane, I saw light dancing on Lake Superior, thousands of metres below. I thought that *we*—everyone who loves and worries for me—not just *I*, will be okay. On the Camino de Cancer, we must cling to these mysteries.

Caring for the Patient

I wonder about the stories healthcare professionals tell themselves, or are told. What story, for example, might cause my hospital room to be flooded with blinding fluorescent light at the blackest time of the morning—the part of morning I call *night*—and prompt a viciously cheerful, "Good morning, Mr. Galliano, breakfast time!" What narrative of care could possibly trump rest for a post-operative patient, could excuse such a cruel start to a day of pain? When I asked, the response was, "Shift change."

What narratives could possibly rationalize the corralling of patients like cattle in waiting rooms? It is no doubt a story about the physician's precious time being worth much more than mine, a narrative about the doctor being more valuable than the patient. On one occasion, while packed in with the rest of the herd, I let out a low-bawling "Moo." It needed doing. My fellow bovine captives chuckled. Then we went back to chewing our cud and reading golf, financial management, and ancient *Reader's Digest* magazines.

Dr. Sarah Newbery is a family doctor in Marathon. She's a teacher of medical students and a past president of the Ontario College of Family Physicians. Sarah is also a dear friend of ours.

When I was convalescing in Toronto General Hospital after my 2015 surgery, Sarah kept us abreast of goings-on back home. She sent daily e-mail missives that read like a small-town newspaper's social column: news of babies arriving, elders departing, and visitors coming to town. She sent updates on the heaviness of ash berry bunches and how they foretold a snowy winter. She passed along good wishes from mutual friends and neighbours. One morning, Sarah described for us the dancing aurora borealis in the moonless sky the previous night.

One of her e-mails concluded this way: "David, I hope that everyone who is caring for your medical needs understands that they are engaged in an act of love." That is her narrative of care. It is a narrative that reaches back to the earliest days of modern medicine.

In a speech to Harvard medical students on October 21, 1925, the legendary physician and Harvard Medical School professor Dr. Francis Weld Peabody said, "One of the essential qualities of the clinician is interest in humanity *for the secret of the care of the patient is in caring for the patient.*" The italics are mine. That's *the* secret: caring for the patient.

Care for the patient is too often lost amid stress and hustle, in specialization and compartmentalization, in technology-based treatments, in data and statistics. Yet, genuine care for the patient is *the* essential plot to the story of care. Professionalism and expertise don't add up to a hill of beans if the provider doesn't care—if he or she doesn't understand that their work is, first and foremost, the embodiment of love for another human being.

How different might our medical system be if it were structured in ways that embodied love? If each and every person working in that system understood they were engaged in caring for the patient?

I know, everyone from the surgeon to the nurse to the social worker and the cleaner feels stretched, overworked, and underappreciated. But I don't think our friend Sarah was talking about some kind of time-sucking, romantic, squishy, poetic, dewy-eyed love. I think she meant a demanding, physical, practical kind of love. A self-giving love of blood and bone and breath and soul. A love that never loses sight of the fact that this patient could be my daughter, my father, or my lover—a multi-storied, complex human being, a living miracle. A love that embraces the honour of bearing witness to another's suffering.

Before being discharged from the hospital, I am usually asked to complete a patient care evaluation questionnaire. Here's a suggestion for improving those questionnaires: Don't just ask about how my care was *in general*. Generally speaking, my experience-of-care scores are in the upper-medium range, say eight out of ten, in all categories. But in actuality, the care I received has often been exceptional and occasionally abysmal. The two average out to a high-medium score, but that doesn't tell the whole story.

In addition to the usual questions, I would like to be asked, "When did you experience genuine *care*?" or "Who seemed to care for you as a human being?" or "Who seemed to understand that they are engaged in an act of love?" I would answer:

- the man who cleaned my bathroom and was whistling while he worked but stopped and apologized for disturbing my rest. When I said, "No, don't stop, it makes me feel good," he kept on whistling and then stood for a moment at the end of my bed to finish the song.

- the surgeon who suggested we meet by video for a follow-up appointment. He understood how difficult it is make the two-day trip to Toronto from Marathon after surgery.

- the nurse who rested her hand on mine while her colleague winched the long drain from beneath the incision in my thigh. There was no medical necessity for that touch, but it alleviated some of my pain.

- the admission clerk who asked me how I was feeling when I arrived at 5:00 a.m. for surgery. I told her I was hungry, anxious, and dying for a coffee. She stopped what she was doing for the five seconds it took to listen and said she would make sure there was a coffee waiting for me when I woke up.

- the nurse who spoke softly and reassuringly as I fought my way up from anaesthesia after surgery. She touched my ear. She said, "Maybe we should start with a sip of water, before coffee."

- the MRI technician who noticed the novel I was reading and recommended one he had loved.

- the staff who remembered my name, pronounced it correctly (not "Mr. Galliano"), and told me their names.

These people deserved more than a medium-to-high ranking. For patients, there is healing in small, humanizing gestures. There is care for the patient in them. I think that is the kind of embodied love Sarah was writing about.

Yes, We Have No Raisins Today

But for the light seeping in from the hallway, the hospital room is dark. It is the second day, post-surgery. My body lies on the bed, dumb as clay, nauseated, aching, and stinking.

Meanwhile, my mind is busy. *Do I need more pain meds? Did I actually hear the nurse say that the guy in the next bed should be in isolation? How hairy will the flap of flesh transplanted from my thigh to my forehead get? Will the titanium mesh used to replace skull-bone create problems in airports? Am I having a stroke? A clot? What's my blood pressure? I need prunes.* I could go on. Believe me, my brain did.

I tried to calm my thoughts with a relaxation meditation, starting with my toes. I ended up drifting away and restarting at least five times—never getting past my knees—before throwing in the contemplative towel.

Then I remembered the *Meditation for Beginners* CD in Pearl's laptop. Squinting through my bulky eyelids,

I found the audio player and the earbuds and booted up the CD. I scrunched the thin pillow beneath my head, ready to welcome the guidance of mindfulness expert Jon Kabat-Zinn.

Pan flutes and chiming prayer bells flowed into my ears. Peacefulness descended like a flannel quilt.

"Mindfulness has to do with paying attention to the things we don't ordinarily pay attention to," began Sensei Kabat-Zinn.

Ah, yes. Take me there, Jon.

"Let's have some raisins on hand," he continued.

Raisins?

"We're just going to take one of them and bring it up towards the face for closer inspection. Just drink it in through the eyes, as if you've never seen one of these before, maybe even forgetting that it's called a raisin."

I don't have a raisin. In the dark, I pat the table, feeling around for a substitute. Who has a raisin just lying around waiting for Kabat-Zinn to tell them to drink it in? And newsflash: you can't drink a raisin in through your eyes, especially if your eyes are swollen shut. This is stupid.

". . . noticing its surface features, its colour, shape, as you turn it in your hand. Seeing whether there are any unique features to it."

The peaceful tone and cadence of Kabat-Zinn's voice starts to grate on my nerves. I cross my arms across my chest, and the IV needle jabs into my wrist. The pain is strangely consoling.

Kabat-Zinn barrels ahead. "As I am doing it, I notice a little circular scarring at one end which, of course, you'll know is the equivalent of our bellybutton."

Oh, for the love of . . .

I shift in the bed, setting off a fresh jolt of electric pain and nausea, skip to the next guided meditation: "Mindfulness Breathing." Good. I fold the stingy pillow in half and stuff it back under my neck.

"Let's take the same quality of attention we just brought to eating the raisin," Kabat-Zinn begins.

I don't have a f—ing raisin, Jon! Yes! We have no raisins today! With or without bellybuttons!

I close the laptop, toss the earbuds onto the table, re-cross my arms over my fetid hospital gown, and savour a fresh stab to the wrist. Fortunately, it's not time for the nurse to check my vitals: my blood pressure is probably through the roof.

Sometimes, on the Camino de Cancer, it's difficult to be contemplative. And sometimes, we just don't have any raisins to drink in with our eyes. Sometimes, it's all we can do to just be present, where we are, accepting our fears and anxious minds. Maybe later, if we're lucky, we can even laugh at ourselves a little.

Reunion

On her way down to the hospital food court for supper, Pearl ran into Bev Welsh at the elevator. Bev didn't notice Pearl. She pushed the down button and studied the lit numbers above the door.

"Bev?" Pearl asked. Bev stared blankly for a couple of heartbeats. It had been nearly forty years since our lives intersected. Pearl and Bev were miles from the city where we met, and we were all bewildered by medical treatments. It takes a moment for the mind to cover those distances.

Bev and her husband, Bill, were our youth group leaders in Windsor. Young parents of two babies, they devoted themselves to our group of nearly seventy suburban teenagers. It was the 1970s—the heydays of mainline Protestantism.

One evening, leading up to Christmas 1975, Bill and I set out in his blue Ford station wagon en route to the Woolco department store to make a few last-minute toy purchases for the church's charity hampers. The plan was to pick Pearl up on the way. I was fifteen years old and deeply infatuated with Pearl. Bill had noticed. "Are you going to ask her out? You might as well get it over with," he advised. "If she says 'no,' at least you know where you stand."

Inside the store, he taunted me with meaningful glances and encouraging winks. Our shopping completed, Bill, not so subtly, backed the car into Pearl's parent's driveway. He stared straight ahead and said, "I'll just wait here, David. You should walk Pearl to the door."

At the back door, beneath the porch light, I blurted, "Do you want to go out with me?"

This is where Pearl's and my recollections of that night diverge. Pearl claims that she responded enthusiastically, "Yes!" And that we went inside for tea.

I, on the other hand, remember her saying, "Sure, why not?" Then she left me standing outside, happy as a puppy.

Back in the car, Bill chuckled and shook his formidable head when I told him Pearl's response to my declaration of affection. On the drive to my house, he repeated it several times, "Sure, why not," trying it out with various inflections of his voice.

Four decades later, on the sixth floor of Toronto General Hospital, Pearl and Bev found themselves standing side by side at the elevator doors. Bill was recovering from prostate surgery. Across the lobby, I was recovering from another rearranging of my face. What are the odds?

Later, Bill came over to my room. He looked solid, in spite of the post-surgical walker propping him up. His grin and mischievous sparkle were as bright and warm as ever. He stood at the end of my bed, inquiring about my health and waving off my concerns about his own well-being. A splotch of blood stained the front of his hospital gown.

"Sit down, Bill," I said.

"I'm fine," he said, and then, "Maybe, I will sit a little."

We reminisced, and marvelled at the long odds of running into one other in a Toronto hospital after so many years. Pearl and I recounted our competing narratives of that night when I first asked her out. I hoped that Bill would settle finally the dispute in my favour, but he just smiled. We told Bev and Bill how instrumental they were in shaping our lives. We did not remark upon the soft tears that wet Bill's cheeks. What was there to say?

These unanticipated reunions on the Camino de Cancer—made pure and true and vulnerable by hospital gowns and suffering—are like the discovery of small, polished, and forgotten stones we've carried in our pockets, memories of our youth. We are surprised to find that they have been there all along, that we have carried them all these years for just this moment.

Take Up Your Pallet and Walk

*W*e started walking. Walking might be too grand a term for the shuffling, walker-assisted circuits I'm making around the head and neck ward. The scabbing incision—snaking twenty inches up from above my knee—flares with each step. The "milking" drain is safety-pinned to the gown. The skin harvested from my thigh is sewed to my forehead, where the bone of my brow has been replaced with titanium mesh. Rimmed by fine black sutures, the flesh flap looks like a large gob of lard. A drain dribbles blood and something else down the side of my face. A knob of black scab bulges from the bridge of my nose beneath my brow. My left eyelid is swollen closed like a fat, sated leech.

On the post-surgical head and neck ward, my appearance is by no means extraordinary. I've started to think of it as the "little shop of horrors." We limp like zombies, with slabs of pale flesh—harvested from our backs, legs, or arms—sewn to our faces, necks, and across the tops of our heads. Hair springs up around our wounds like weeds on a sidewalk.

There's the persistent wheezing of the freshly tracheotomized and the wet suctioning of their windpipes. "Good for you, Mr. Cuzco, you're doing fine," says a nurse to one of the other patients. "Look at that: your discharge was all dark brown last night, and today it's foamy pink. You're doing great!"

Our wounds are likely no more gruesome than those on other surgical wards, but rather than being tucked away demurely beneath hospital gowns, ours are on display in all their gory glory.

We have become a community of sorts, familiar with one another's fleshly pain, anxiety, and shame. We nod in passing and smile—that is, if we still have jaws and lips with which to smile.

Two mornings in a row, the man across the hall has dressed in anticipation of being discharged. He says his brother is on his way to pick him up. He doesn't know why his brother hasn't come. Some suffering is of the body, and some is of the waiting heart.

Down the hall, a young woman, her bony back turned to the door, perches on the edge of her bed. She faces the window. The window admits a grey autumn light and reflects her misshapen features.

An elderly Sri Lankan woman sits and waits beside her husband's bed. He has not regained consciousness from his surgery two days ago. Each time I pass, we give each other the thumbs up. She cannot speak English, and I cannot speak Sinhalese or Tamil.

A nurse makes his way around the ward, poking his head into each room to announce, "Blue Jays versus Rangers, big screen, 4:00 p.m. in the visitors' lounge." It's game five—do or die—of the 2015 American League Division Series in the race for the World Series championship.

With little else on our schedules and hungry for a win of any kind, we balance our surgically rearranged heads and necks on our shoulders and slipper our way down to the lounge, rearranging the vinyl and chrome chairs for optimum viewing.

The Texas Rangers lead by one until the sixth inning, when the Blue Jays tie the game. Then, the Jays score four times to the Rangers' one in the seventh, and after two scoreless innings, the Jays win the game. The lounge erupts with feeble and wincing sounds of joy.

I look around the room. The man waiting for his brother is there. The Sri Lankan woman—her thumb raised in my direction—is there, too, along with the young woman with the slender back, her face turned for all to see. All of us are united in this space by suffering and by victory. The moment mystically elevates us and erases what seemed gruesome, ugly. What is revealed instead is our humanity—imperfect, vulnerable, and beautiful. It's as though a bright light shines from each soul.

Meal Tray Communion

*I*t is Thanksgiving, and I am thankful in spite of it all. In spite of the flesh-flap and the titanium mesh. In spite of the excruciating pain of having a forty-centimetre drain winched from beneath my knee-to-thigh incision. You know the list: the doctors and nurses; my friends and family who visit; my beloved Pearl and our children; the food and clean sheets; and the beauty of life itself.

I'm genuinely grateful.

Really.

I'm also feeling sorry for myself. Here it is, Thanksgiving, and I'm shuffling the halls of the hospital, trailing my intravenous pole. I'm in pain. Body and soul.

And I'm feeling jealous of everyone who's tucking into a turkey dinner and enjoying the warm glow of familial companionship. And of Pearl, my mom, and my dear friend, Keith Reynolds, who have crossed University Avenue to the

Swiss Chalet for a dinner of chicken, stuffing, cranberry sauce, and potatoes. How self-pitying is that?

By the time *my* dinner arrives, Keith and Mom are on their way home. Pearl is at my bedside. She positions the table over the bed. I push the button to raise the back of it and poke a finger through a venting hole on the plastic lid covering my food. There's a mash of something red and white. It may have been lasagna when it emerged from some subterranean industrial kitchen. That is before it was trucked to the loading dock downstairs. There's a vegetable. Are those carrots? There's tea. There's a little dish of pine-apple. It appears to be fresh, not canned. Be still my heart.

There's a hard, white bun sealed in cellophane. There's a half-cup of juice in a plastic container with a tinfoil lid. I lift the container closer to my right eye—the good one. Grape juice. Heretofore, juices had arrived predictably: orange on the morning tray; apple on the lunch and evening trays. That reliable pattern is shattered by grape, and it seems like a minor miracle.

I'm a preacher and a cradle Christian. To me, a bun and grape juice is Christ's call to the table. It's as reflexive as standing when a hymn is announced or bowing my head to pray. Holding the juice cup in one hand and the bun in the other, I say to Pearl, "We can have communion." I mean it as a little joke, but the words catch in my throat. My eyes spill over.

I finish my lasagna and savour the pineapple. I eat all of it because I'm hungry, and because even in my self-pitying funk, I know there are too many people who would trade plates with me in an instant. I'm privileged in ways that embarrass me.

Pearl goes down the hall to refill my cup with water and ice. While she is gone, I clear the blue plastic tray of detritus, plates, and packaging. I spread a clean white tissue on it, tear open the bun bag with my teeth, and peel back the foil lid of the juice cup. I centre them on the tissue, on top of the tray. When Pearl returns, she sits on the edge of the bed—the elements between us.

I repeat the story of Jesus' last meal—how he broke the bread and poured the wine, and asked his friends to remember him when they ate and drank. We say a prayer, naming the things for which we are grateful. We break and eat the dry bun, and wash it down with grape juice. I don't know if Pearl is crying; my own eyes are too flooded with tears to see. Tears of gratitude for a bun and a cup of grape juice— for Jesus and his friends who I have come to know in those unremarkable elements.

The communion of saints—living and dead—gather round to hold and heal us.

Meanwhile, my roommate is vomiting in the bathroom. The sound of it grounds me, allowing my puny sufferings to be woven together with the far greater sufferings of the world and carry the remembrance of Jesus' own suffering in my body. Paradoxically, my small bit of suffering helps me to feel closer to joy than I have felt all day. I'm grateful for all the Sundays when I ate bread and drank juice, and it meant nothing to me. Each one of those Sundays was training for days like this.

Wolves, I Was Attacked by Wolves

"*W*hat happened to your face?" Kids, especially little boys, just blurt it out. They can't help asking. They stare up at me, mouths agape. Sometimes they are sufficiently oppressed by good manners to whisper it to a parent, "What happened to his face?" Their parents are mortified.

"*H*ey," I reassure their mom or dad, "enquiring minds want to know."

After all, I have two steak-sized slabs of flesh sewn to my face. They were relocated there—beautifully so, from a surgical perspective—from other parts of my body by a world-class plastic surgeon. *Plastic* surgery, please note, is not the same as *cosmetic* surgery. If you google "difference between plastic and cosmetic surgery," you might well find a photo of me next to a photo of Joan Rivers. Surgery has slowed my cancer. It has not made me better looking.

Unlike children, adults pretend not to notice the disfigurement that is as plain as the nose on my face. They try valiantly to maintain eye contact, or gaze into middle-space over my shoulder, unsuccessfully willing their eyes to not notice the elephant in the room, located on my face.

When a little kid asks me what happened to my face, I crouch down to offer them a closer inspection of my flesh-flaps. "Go ahead, you can touch it if you want. It doesn't hurt." And they often run their fingers across my forehead or give it a poke. I wink, look over my left shoulder and then the right, as if preparing to cross a dangerous street together. The street is called "Fact Versus Metaphor Drive." I whisper, "Wolves." I pause, to heighten the drama. "I was attacked by wolves."

The little boy or girl looks at me sideways. A co-conspiring smile flickers on their lips. "Really?" they ask, ready to cross the street with me. "Wolves?"

"Oh, yes," I say. I spin a tale of snapping and snarling wolves felling me like a moose calf on a frozen lake. I mimic their sharp fangs with my teeth and their claws with my curled fingers. I growl and snap and howl and yip. I re-enact a fierce battle. I demonstrate how I broke the wolves' jaws by prying them open with my bare hands. How I kicked them with my boots and swung them over my head by their bushy tails and flung them against the trunks of trees. I am made breathless by the telling.

"Not really," says the child, secretly hoping that it might be true.

At about this point, an appalled parent disrupts the game. "He was *not*," they reprimand me, "attacked by wolves!" They point a quivering finger in my direction. "You had better be at our house at bedtime tonight, mister."

Chastened, I tell the child, "It wasn't wolves. It was cancer." Which is not particularly helpful to an eight-year-old. He or she usually responds with disappointment, "I know."

I have lost count of the number of surgeries I've endured. I've had the two major surgeries I've already described. (My definition of "major surgery": surgery done to us. My definition of "minor surgery": surgery done to somebody else.) They left long grizzly scars down my back and my thigh in addition to the ones on my face that fascinate children. I am also now irreparably double-visioned due to the detaching and reattaching of optical muscle during the second surgery.

Radiation therapy left me with numerous permanent side effects. The short list includes: permanent loss of one tear gland, necessitating the application of eye drops every thirty to sixty minutes for the *rest of my life*; one cataract surgery; two detached retina surgeries (including, in one case, having my eyeball slit to remove injected silicone, without the benefit of anaesthesia); and the blowout of a radiation-hardened blood vessel in my brain, causing a stroke. The eyelid of the eye with no tear gland drifts open while I sleep. So I tape it closed at night; otherwise, I wake up feeling like it was poked with a hot, pointed stick.

The psychosocial effect of cancer treatment has been no bowl of cherries either. One of the ophthalmologists I saw—to cite just one random example—schedules all his patients for 9:00 a.m. Patients are corralled in the waiting room and forced to watch a "*Home Alone 2*" video looping over and over on the television until it's their turn to be seen.

Trying to strike up a friendly conversation, when it was finally my turn, I said to this doctor, "Wow, you seem really busy."

"Yes, I wish I could have one of those baggage conveyer belts, like at the airport," he replied. "The patients could just roll by on it." I laughed before realizing that he wasn't joking.

On another occasion, I was riding a post-op opioid nag and trying to pee in a plastic bottle under the bed sheet. At that exact moment, an army of surgical residents and interns surrounded my bed, snapping on blue rubber gloves. The head resident, without looking up from his clipboard, bellowed, "Hello, Mr. Galliano. How are you doing?"

"Well," I smiled dopily, and referencing their interruption, I said, "I am having a little trouble peeing."

Clearly a man of action, he shouted at the nurse, "Get Mr. Galliano some Flomax." They snapped off the rubber gloves, scattering them on the floor and on me as they marched out. *Our work here is done!* It took two days of overflowing plastic bottles and bedwetting to convince the nurses that, contrary to doctor's order for Flomax, I was not in need of urinary assistance.

Don't try to joke with the head resident. Trust me.

On balance, I've had excellent medical care. Most of the personnel who treated me were highly skilled and beautifully human. I love them—and not just in a Stockholm syndrome sort of way. But cancer treatment, by the very nature of the beast, involves a lot of violence.

So when a kid asks me, "What happened to your face?" I can either regale them with tales of clinical brutalization, or I can tell them I was attacked by wolves. Both narratives are, in their own way, true. There is a cure in one and healing

119

in the other. The one about wolves is a hell of a lot more fun. And kids know all about wolves. They confront them every day.

Not Forgetting

*W*e arrive at Mecca or Graceland or Lourdes. We rest on the steps of the cathedral in Santiago. Pilgrimages often end with an unshakable certainty that we are changed and will never be the same. Certain that we won't forget the wisdom gained, the beauty perceived, or the bonds of love created on the journey.

It's been two years since my last Camino de Cancer, and I forget sometimes. Forget the bread and the juice and how it quenches my deepest thirsts and hungers. Forget the beauty revealed by brokenness. Forget to live simply and slowly. Forget to notice the miracle of life, all of life. Forget kindness and gentleness, my own and others. Forget the mysterious encounters with the presence of the crucified Christ through suffering.

So it is good every now and then to flip through the photos taken, or the diary kept on the journey. Pin a map to the wall and trace the route travelled with your forefinger.

Dim the lights and put on a slideshow for your friends. Revisit the stories, like I have with you. So I don't forget.

If we are awake, all the pathways of the soul are open to us. We experience each of them by just being alive. The *Via Positiva, Via Creativa, Via Transformativa,* and *Via Negativa.* No one chooses the *Via Negativa.* Sooner or later, it just shows up on your doorstep, an unwelcome travelling companion bearing difficult gifts.

Postscript:

It's Good to Be Here

These are some stories I know. They are stories I've been told and ones I tell about cancer, illness, and suffering. That's all we are: stories. Fantasy author Patrick Rothfuss puts it this way in his 2007 novel, *The Name of The Wind*: "It's like everyone tells a story about themselves inside their head. Always. All the time. That story makes you who you are. We build ourselves out of that story." Other people tell the stories that end up in our head too. The stories that create us and by which we create the world are multidimensional, complex, and evolving. The narratives we tell and the metaphors we use about cancer shape our experience of illness. Some stories can be healing. Some can even cure.

It is difficult but essential to tell narratives that understand suffering as part of life. It is also helpful to distinguish between the interwoven natures of cure and of healing in our narratives.

The narratives people kept telling me—about blame and battle—were not healing. They left me feeling sick and ashamed.

The stories I find healing are narratives about temples, treasure, pilgrimage, wolves, and love. They help me talk about cancer in ways that feel meaningful and humanizing. I tried to redeem my cancer—find the gift in the unwelcome blessing—through metaphors about scars, light, vulnerability, *caminos*, violence, and caring. Those metaphors and many, many others create me and my understanding of what it is to be human. Through them, I come to know and love the world.

Since I began telling people my stories about cancer and health care, they have told me theirs.

"It is like mountain climbing—hard, dangerous work," said one person, "but the view can be breathtaking at times."

"Cancer weighed me down," another person told me. "I was so depressed and felt alone. It was like I was carrying this heavy backpack on my back. The pack was full of my worries and shame and fear. Then I started to let friends and family help me carry it. A counsellor helped me look inside it to see what I could take out and set down to lighten the load. Especially the shame."

In her 2015 book *Malignant Metaphor*, science writer Alanna Mitchell asks: "What if we talked about cancer as a dance instead of a war? What if we could hear some music in it? What would it sound like? What if we could take turns leading and being led by illness toward healing?"

At the opening of the Health Quality Ontario Conference in 2016, president and CEO Dr. Joshua Tepper described healthcare as a puzzle. "It requires having all the pieces and fitting them together to create a whole picture." I think the metaphors and narratives we use to talk about cancer and illness are essential parts of that puzzle. When we add those pieces we begin to see something new.

Last week, it was very cold here in Marathon, the kind of cold that makes our wood-framed houses pop. Our cars moan when they start. Windshields crack of their own voli-tion. The snow is dry and squeaks like Styrofoam underfoot. We keep an eye out for bursting pipes. I waited until after lunch, when the temperature had climbed to -20°C, to go for a ski. Bundled in multiple layers of fleece and nylon, I set out on the trails.

The ineffectual but brilliant December sun slanted through the dense woods, turning the snow to diamonds. It turned the snow-shadows cradled in the spruce boughs purple. The thin, skeletal birch and poplar limbs were outlined in white. I stopped and watched the puffs of my steaming breath. I removed a mitten to quickly run a thumb across the frosted lenses of my sunglasses and scrape some ice from my beard.

I could hear the flap of a raven's wings as it dropped down from the crown of a tree. A woodpecker hammered in the distance. In the whisper of breeze, a peel of birch bark rattled against the trunk of its tree. And I thought, *It's good to be here.*

That is a narrative I'm telling these days, a story I'm trying to live.

Above all else, it is a narrative of gratitude. Gratitude for a long list of people who inhabit and serve in the medical system, for family and friends and strangers who have been my faithful companions. Gratitude for the miracle of life, even for the unwelcome blessings of suffering. Gratitude for the infinite universe, expansive beyond my comprehension. Gratitude for my peculiar, perfect place in it.

It is good to be here.

Thank You

Thank you to the countless medical professionals who accompanied me on the Camino. There are too many to list them all. An exceptional few, however, must be named: Doctors Gilbert and O'Sullivan—whose librettist names are best said in tandem—for their fierce curiosity and superstar skills; and doctors Sarah Newbery and Eli Orrantia, who are great family physicians and even better family friends. Faithfull companions in The United Church of Canada, who welcomed my leadership when I was weak. Editor David Wilson, who took a scalpel to the original manuscript—it was painful, but it needed doing. Rev. Dr. Nancy Lane who, as my spiritual director, helped me learn to listen with care to my life and my dreams. Above all, I am grateful for Jeremiah, Naomi, and Pearl, who continue to endure with love my telling of stories, over and over and over.

Questions for Reflection

INTRODUCTION

David quotes Thomas King, "The truth about stories is, that is all we are."

What are the stories you were told as a child that have shaped you? Who told them?

Share or journal some of the stories you've heard about illness and suffering.

PART ONE

In "A Scar Near My Temple," there is an invitation to listen to the wisdom of the body.

When or how have you experienced a "body-mind connection"?

For David, 2 Corinthians 4:7—"We have this treasure in earthen vessels"—became a touchstone. Have you experienced the treasure within vulnerability or seen it around you? Are there sacred texts in your own religious or secular tradition that are touchstones for you?

Brené Brown says, "Vulnerability is the birthplace of love, belonging, joy, courage, empathy, and creativity." Why do you think we are so uncomfortable with vulnerability—our own or others?

Think about a time you felt afraid. Share or journal about how you respond to fear.

The chapter "Welcoming the Wound" ends with a prayer. Try praying it quietly to yourself or reading it together if you are gathered in a group.

In "Blame and Battle," David describes common narratives we tell about illness in general and cancer in particular. Have these stories been helpful to you? Have you told them yourself? How have they been encouraging or comforting for you? How have they been harmful?

Darkness. Do you have any positive feelings about darkness? Share or write about stories associated with darkness.

What images of God have shaped your spirituality? David encountered the presence of the God who *tabernacles*—makes a home—in what is weak and vulnerable (in a teenager on the subway). How do feel about a God who is vulnerable and weak?

"Sang Chul knows that the Great Mystery sometimes calls us to lead in ways we would rather not." Can you think of other examples of leaders who felt called to lead in ways they would have preferred not to lead? Have there been times when life has called you to places you would rather not go? How did you react?

Read out loud (or sing if you know the tune) Libby Roderick's lyrics, "How could anyone tell you / You were anything less than beautiful." If you are in a group, take turns reading or singing the lyrics to one person at a time. How does it feel having these words said/sung to you?

"Joy & Woe are woven fine / A Clothing for the soul divine," wrote William Blake. Share your own stories about joy and woe woven fine. Do you agree with David that we live in a culture that sees suffering as an aberration? A failure? A source of shame? Why or why not?

In a blog post—"Singing in a Strange Land"—David writes about feelings of despair. He shares two very different pastoral comments that were made to the post. Both are encouraging in their own way. Which one would comfort you more? Why?

Have you heard the cliché, "Where there is life there is hope" before? In what context did you hear it? David turns it around: "Where there is hope there is life." Agree? Disagree?

Have you or someone you know experienced a physical, spiritual, or emotional event that changed your/their appearance? Share or journal about that event.

David rejected help from a stranger who telephoned while he was spending time with his son, Jeremiah. What are your thoughts about that? Might he have missed an opportunity? What would you have said to the caller?

Are there times in your own life when you experienced healing but not a cure, or a cure but not healing? Share or journal about those times.

Are you familiar with sacred texts—the Torah, Koran, Gospel, etc.—in which sudden healings or cures take place? What do you make of those stories? How has curing and healing happened in your own life—suddenly or un-suddenly?

Write down five ways in which you are remarkable. If you are in a group, name aloud for yourself, or for each other the ways you/they are remarkable.

PART TWO

Have you ever made a geographic, physical pilgrimage? Where to? Share or write about how/if it impacted on you—spiritually? Emotionally? Relationally? Physically?

Which of the four spiritual paths—*positiva, creativa, transformativa,* or *negativa*—have been most significant in your life?

David says in "Eli Comes Calling" that, "Stoicism is my usual first response—my go-to in fearful times. Denial and bargaining aren't my way." What is your first response to bad or frightening news? Can you trace that response back to a story you've been told, or to an earlier time in your life?

Raphael visits David's father in a dream. Have you ever had a supernatural experience like that? What meaning was in it for you? For example, did you find forgiveness or healing or encouragement or guidance or something else in it? Share that experience with your group or record it for yourself.

"I cope by going inside myself. When I'm sick, I lack the energy to host the questions and the anxieties of those who love me." How do you cope with illness or suffering? How do you respond to those who are worried about you?

"Dr. Francis Weld Peabody said . . . 'the secret of the care of the patient is in *caring for the patient.*'" What has been your experience of being cared for or not cared for by healthcare professionals? How did it make a difference?

Do you meditate or practise mindfulness or some other form of contemplation? If you do, what frustrations and gifts have come to you through your practice? What other ways bring you peacefulness in difficult times?

Pearl meets Bev at the elevators. Share some stories of unexpected meetings? How do you interpret those experiences—serendipity? Fluke? Miracle? Has your understanding of that unexpected encounter changed over time? How? Do you share this story with others?

"Take Up Your Pallet and Walk" ends with the following: "What is revealed instead is our humanity—imperfect, vulnerable, and beautiful. It's as though a bright light shines from each soul." When have you seen this sort of vulnerable beauty, the light of humanity? Was it your own or someone else's?

"I'm grateful," David writes, "for all the Sundays when I ate bread and drank juice, and it meant nothing to me." Rituals are, in part, like training is for athletes. They prepare us for events when strength or courage or comfort is needed. Are there rituals—religious or secular—in which you find meaning in difficult times?

Wolves and cancer treatments: David says both stories are true. Think about trauma or suffering in your life. Write or tell a children's story or a metaphor that describes that experience.

If you've been on a geographic pilgrimage, what memories do you continue to revisit and share with others? Likewise, if you've been on a spiritual or emotional *camino*, what memories do you continue to revisit and share with others? Reflect on the differences, if there are any.

"Since I began telling other people my stories about cancer and health care," writes David, "they have told me theirs." What narratives about illness or suffering speak to you? When do you find yourself thinking, *It's good to be here*?

About the Author

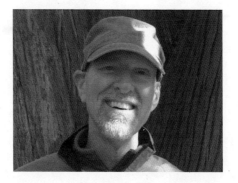

Photo Credit: Jeremiah Giuliano

David Giuliano is an award-winning writer of essays, stories, and poems. His book *Postcards from the Valley: Encounters with Fear, Faith and God* was a Canadian bestseller.

Visit www.davidgiuliano.ca to learn more about the author, to schedule an online book club conversation, or to extend an invitation to speak at your event.

Printed in Canada